Knee Replacement Secrets is an invaluable resource for anyone feeling the fear and uncertainty of surgery. It offers reassurance and guidance for those facing this life-changing decision. My own experience with Dr. Sinha and Conformis has been transformative, and I share my gratitude every chance I get. This book will undoubtedly help others navigate their journey with confidence.

—Dave L.

Knee Replacement Secrets is a must-read for anyone facing knee challenges or considering surgery. It provides clear, transparent guidance on what to expect, empowering readers to make informed decisions about their knee health. Diana's personal journey and emphasis on early knee care resonated with me, giving me the confidence to stop powering through pain and seek medical guidance. This book is an invaluable resource for anyone navigating knee issues and looking for clarity on their next steps—or making the decision to go bionic!

—Charlyn R.

Diana Braun has been a tremendous help to me in my recovery after my total knee replacement. It has been so wonderful to be able to talk to someone who had recently been through what I was going through. I always enjoy talking to her on the phone or texting with her, and her weekly/biweekly recovery guides have been extremely helpful.

She has helped me to understand that everything I've been feeling and going through is normal. And, at the same time, she's made it clear that everyone's healing journey is different. She's very empathetic and understanding, and she's truly a great coach! I know this would have been a much harder journey without her. Thanks, Diana!

—Janet K.

I highly recommend this book to anyone considering knee surgery—and keep it close during recovery! Diana's personal experience, from deciding on surgery to navigating recovery, is invaluable for those facing the same journey. Her reminder that "we are not all in the same boat, but we are in the same storm" would have been especially helpful to me during my own process.

She reminds us that healing isn't always linear. Even after nearly a year of recovery, I needed to hear that. While many say, "six months to a year" is typical, this book emphasizes that everyone's healing timeline is different, which was comforting during my own ups and downs.

The book's structure is excellent—Diana's firsthand experience paired with Dr. Sinha's medical insights strikes the perfect balance between personal and professional perspectives. After reading it through, I found myself returning to the recovery section for both encouragement and a reality check!

—Jeanne M.

This book is an invaluable resource for anyone facing knee replacement surgery. The start-to-finish explanation of the journey helps patients prepare pre-op and navigate the ups and downs of recovery with confidence.

One of the best aspects is how it normalizes the recovery process. Each time I revisit sections of the book, I feel reassured that my experience is typical and that recovery takes time.

I love the balance between Diana's empathetic, personal storytelling and Dr. Sinha's clear medical analysis. Their combined perspectives make the book both engaging and informative, blending real-world patient experiences with expert medical insights—the secret sauce that makes this guide so effective.

—A.J.

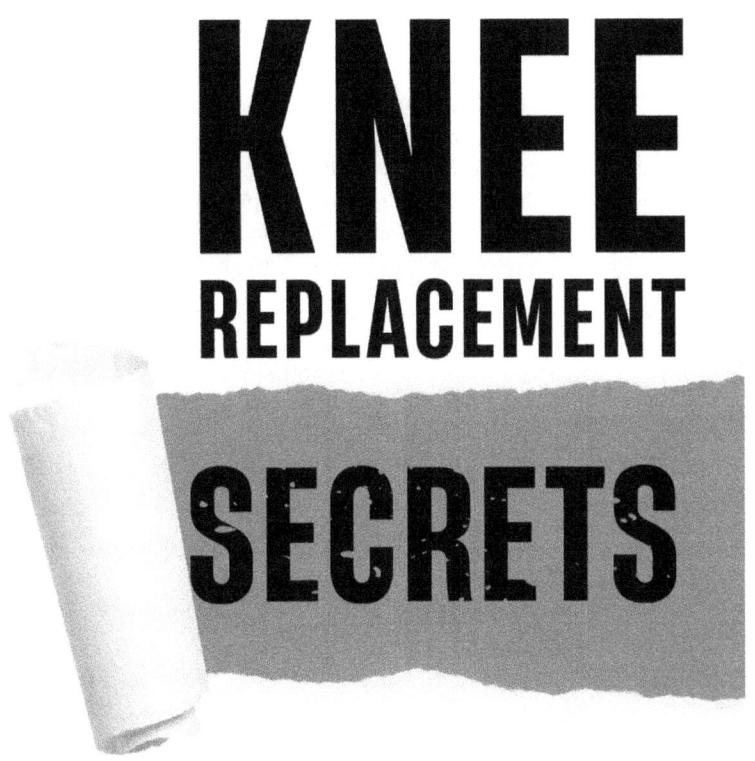

KNEE REPLACEMENT SECRETS

Everything You "Knee'd" to Know About Avoiding, Preparing For, and Recovering From Arthroplasty by an Actual Patient and an Orthopedic Surgeon

**DIANA BRAUN, CHPC,
& RAJ SINHA, MD, PHD, FAAOS**

KNEE REPLACEMENT SECRETS

Everything You "Knee'd" to Know About Avoiding, Preparing For, and Recovering From Arthroplasty by an Actual Patient and an Orthopedic Surgeon

Copyright © 2025. Diana Braun, CHPC, and Raj Sinha, MD, PhD, FAAOS. All rights reserved. No part of this publication may be reproduced, distributed, or transmitted in any form or by any means, including photocopying, recording, or other electronic or mechanical methods, without the prior written permission of the publisher, except in the case of brief quotations embodied in critical reviews and certain other noncommercial uses permitted by copyright law.

For permission requests, speaking inquiries, and bulk order purchase options, visit thekneezone.com.

The Knee Zone, LLC
P.O. Box 1204
Belton, TX 76513

TheKneeZone.com

Book Design by Transcendent Publishing
Editing by Lori Lynn Enterprises

ISBN: 979-8-9928630-4-8

Disclaimer: The information provided in this book was written to provide helpful information on how to delay, prepare for, and recover from Total Knee Replacements. It should not be considered as personal medical advice. This book is not meant to be used, nor should it be used, to diagnose or treat any medical condition. You have not become a patient of Raj Sinha, MD, PhD, or a client of Diana Braun, CHPC, by reading this book, and you should consult with your physician regarding your medical care. For diagnosis or treatment of any medical problem, please consult a physician.

Raj Sinha and Diana Braun are not responsible for any specific health or allergy needs that may require medical supervision and are not liable for any damages or negative consequences from any treatment, action, application, or preparation to any person reading or following the information in this book. As with any new exercise program, you should consult your doctor or surgeon for approval before commencing. Please consult your doctor immediately if you feel unwell, dizzy, or experience shortness of breath or chest pain while exercising. References are provided for informational purposes only and do not constitute endorsement of any websites or other sources of information.

Readers should be aware that the QR codes and websites listed in this book may change.

"Better, Faster, Stronger."

—**Bionic Woman**

CONTENTS

Dedication xi
Doctors Recommend Knee Replacement Secrets xiii
The Bridge to Freedom from Pain 1
Is Putting It Off Putting You at Risk? 13
    I'm Too Busy for Surgery 15
What You Knee'd to Know When Considering Total Knee Replacement 19
    What You "Knee'd" to Know Before Your Bionic Upgrade 21
Preparing for Surgery 43
    Pre-Hab for Knee Replacement 45
    The Big Bionic Upgrade Day 63
Let the Healing Journey Begin 75
    Weekly Recovery Guide| Weeks 1 & 2 77
    Recovery Guide What To Expect | Weeks 2–4 105
Your Monthly Goals 121
    Months 1 & 2 | Getting Out Into the World 123

Bend and Prosper **141**
   Month 3 | Getting Back to Normal 143

Midway Milestones **151**
   Months 4 & 5 | You're Halfway to Total Healing! . . . 153

Month 6 & Beyond The Homestretch **161**
   Start Saying "YES!" 163

Kicking the Can Down the Road **169**
   Tips on How to Avoid Surgery. 171

Final Thoughts **185**
   Diana's Final Thoughts. 185
   Dr. Sinha Shares the History—and Future—of
      Knee Replacement Surgery. 186

Let's Keep in Touch! **193**

Acknowledgments 195
About the Authors 199
May We Ask a Favor? 201
How to Get More Help 203

DEDICATION

For our "bionic upgraded" friends and family.

DOCTORS RECOMMEND *KNEE REPLACEMENT SECRETS*

Making the decision to undergo knee replacement surgery can be overwhelming. As a Doctor of Physical Therapy, I spend countless hours educating patients on what to expect before, during, and after the procedure. However, there's only so much information that can be covered in a single session. That's why *Knee Replacement Secrets* is such a valuable resource—it provides patients with a comprehensive, easy-to-understand guide to help them feel informed and prepared at every stage of their journey.

Diana Braun and Dr. Raj Sinha have created a book that is not only informative but also engaging and relatable. Diana's firsthand experience as a patient, combined with Dr. Sinha's expert medical perspective, ensures a well-rounded, practical approach.

The book covers essential topics that I emphasize daily, from the importance of maintaining physical therapy exercises to budgeting for post-surgery costs. The authors include key information that is often overlooked, including avoiding excessive activity and the realistic overall timeframe for recovery. The visuals and humor throughout make the content approachable, helping to ease the stress that often comes with this major life decision.

One of the standout points in this book is the emphasis on achieving full knee extension early in recovery—something that is often not a priority at first, yet crucial for long-term mobility, normalizing gait and reducing pain. The discussion on the reality of physical therapy costs, sleeping positions, and even the notes on adhesive allergies highlights just how thorough and thoughtful this guide is.

Knee Replacement Secrets is a must-read for anyone considering or recovering from knee replacement surgery. It empowers patients with knowledge, helping them take control of their recovery with confidence. I will be highly recommending this book to my patients and am excited for the impact it will have on so many lives.

—Lara Herzog, DPT

As a Doctor of Physical Therapy, I had the privilege of reading an advance copy of *Knee Replacement Secrets*, and I can confidently say it is an invaluable resource for anyone navigating the journey of total knee replacement (TKR).

Diana Braun and Dr. Sinha have done an outstanding job creating a thorough, well-written guide that offers both the patient's and the doctor's perspectives. This dual approach provides a unique and balanced view that will undoubtedly bring peace of mind to those considering or undergoing knee replacement surgery.

I found the tips on post-surgery sleep and driving considerations especially beneficial. I also appreciate the emphasis on pre-hab—something I teach my patients as well—and the detailed guidance on preparing for surgery.

Knee Replacement Secrets offers a thorough, practical, and compassionate guide for anyone considering knee replacement surgery. I highly recommend to patients and professionals alike.

—Yana Cheatham, PT, DPT

Knee Replacement Secrets is an excellent resource that I highly recommend. Having had the opportunity to advance-read the book, I can confidently say it offers valuable insights and guidance for those considering knee replacement surgery.

Diana Braun and Dr. Sinha have created a thorough, practical guide that emphasizes the importance of following your surgeon's recommended pathway to recovery, while also acknowledging that there are multiple ways to achieve a good result. Listen to your surgeon and read this book!

—Kipling Sharpe, MD

An exceptional resource for anyone considering or undergoing knee replacement surgery, *Knee Replacement Secrets* corresponds with my experience and the guidance I provide to my patients.

What truly sets this book apart is its unique combination of a patient's perspective and a surgeon's expertise. The clear, easy-to-read format, enhanced with helpful pictures and practical advice, ensures that readers can follow along at every stage of their recovery. The breakdown of timeframes, specific do's and don'ts, and step-by-step instructions for everyday activities like getting in and out of a car or choosing the right chair make this book not only informative but incredibly actionable.

One of the book's standout features is its flexibility: readers can "jump" ahead to the section most relevant to their current stage of recovery, making it easy to navigate and find exactly what they need. This feature, along with the practical tips for managing pain, post-surgery care, and preparation, allows both patients and healthcare providers to focus on recovery rather than spending time explaining the basics.

I highly recommend *Knee Replacement Secrets* to anyone considering knee replacement surgery. Not only does it offer a comprehensive overview of the healing process, but it also sets realistic expectations before, during, and after surgery.

I'm excited to share this book with patients as it's packed with expert advice and actionable tips that will help ensure a smoother, more successful recovery.

—Jon Elbert, PT, DPT, OCS

THE BRIDGE TO FREEDOM FROM PAIN

Chrysteen had always been healthy and active. For decades, she and her husband ran a remodeling business, keeping her on the go. But one day, her knee just started hurting.

Nothing happened to trigger the pain—no injuries or falls. Since her work required significant daily movement, she assumed that giving her knee a break would help. As she neared retirement, she planned to stop remodeling and start writing.

Her dreams of becoming a published author were just over the horizon. Hoping the pain would eventually disappear, she began her new writing career. But the lack of movement didn't seem to help.

Gradually, walking longer distances became more and more difficult, and climbing the stairs in the house was a constant source of pain. Instead of getting better, her knee pain seemed to be getting increasingly worse.

She loved her two-story home and wanted to continue to live there with her husband, so they installed a chair lift on the stairs. They figured it would benefit both of them as time went on. Sure enough, as hoped, the lift immediately eliminated the strain and relieved her knee pain while navigating the stairs.

Later, after she discovered that she had developed osteoarthritis, a chronic disease that causes the cartilage in joints to break down, causing pain, swelling, and stiffness, she began to consider knee replacement surgery. She had the unusual advantage of having a son-in-law who is a knee replacement surgeon, so the topic would often come up during family gatherings.

A turning point came when she and her husband spent a week together on a cruise to Alaska. They planned ahead and decided to bring a walker along, carefully considered the excursions, and ensured ice would be available to ice and elevate her knee each night. But the trip still required lots of walking and standing, and her pain kept escalating. It was both frustrating and exhausting.

After lying awake at night, questions swirling about what to do, she seriously started to consider surgery as an option. Watching her stepdaughter recover from having her knees replaced gave her hope. She got to see someone she was close to with firsthand experience make a full recovery—not only from having one knee replaced but both—and at the same time!

She talked to several people she knew who had had knee replacements, and they were all glad they did it except for one. That one friend had surgery years ago, but he later admitted he didn't do a great job following instructions for physical therapy and ultimately regretted his lack of follow-up.

Since she'd already fought cancer and won that battle, she knew she could set her mind on a successful outcome and achieve it. More than anything, she wanted to get her quality of life back.

She asked all the questions she could think of when she spoke with her surgeon son-in-law about how to prepare, what to expect, and why she might be a good candidate.

She also spoke with her stepdaughter at length about her experience with double knee replacement surgery. Once she felt she could make an informed decision, Chrysteen talked to a local orthopedic surgeon to schedule her bionic upgrade.

Six weeks after surgery, she was able to attend the book launch signing for her newest book. She is currently doing the rehab work and has come to understand that although progress is not linear (each day is up and down), she can appreciate how much she is improving each week.

We haven't mentioned yet that my name is Diana Braun, and Chrysteen is my stepmom. Dr. Sinha is my husband. He and I are the co-founders of The Knee Zone, a community for people like Chrysteen who "knee'd" to know what to expect, how to plan, and what steps to take to bounce back from knee replacement.

Chrysteen learned all sorts of tips and tricks from her knee coaching. She learned how to plan for the big day, her return home, and the weeks that followed.

She graciously read this book, suggested ways to improve the areas that needed further development, and confirmed that the stages of preparation and healing were fairly predictable.

Once Chrysteen discovered a way out of the pain and suffering—a path back to the life she thought she'd lost forever, she knew that was the best decision for her. She learned what most people don't know about knee replacement—that it's not just a surgery, it's a chance to reclaim the life you thought you'd lost. To live without pain. To walk again without wincing. To climb stairs, play with your grandkids, or simply stand up and feel strong.

Knee pain may have brought you here, but there's hope. This book is your answer. It's your roadmap to understanding knee replacement, not just as a procedure but as a bridge to the freedom and joy you deserve.

Who Is Diana Braun?

Before I co-founded The Knee Zone and wrote this book with my husband, I put off having surgery for more than 10 years.

"Please, just a little more time—I have this *one* last trip planned!" That was me in June 2023. I was so excited about the trip my friend and I had planned—a yoga retreat to Italy.

Initially, we booked it for 2020, but the global pandemic forced us to reschedule. Three years later, with the anticipation building for our long-overdue trip, I noticed my knees were getting progressively worse.

A few weeks after I bought my airline tickets, my knee pain went from bad to terrible. Then something new started happening. I was having nightmares. The nightmares got my attention.

I would wake up in a sweat during the middle of the night with my heart pounding and feeling stabbing pain in *both* my knees. This pain was at an entirely new level and certainly concerning, as I hadn't been having nearly the same amount of pain in my left knee as I had in my right.

My husband is a highly talented and experienced joint replacement surgeon. Lucky me, right? I woke him up in the middle of the night, whimpering in pain. I asked if there was anything else we could try so I could still make my trip—please?

He finally found the perfect time to negotiate with me. "Yes, if you promise to get new X-rays and CT scans and schedule your surgery."

Yes, of course, I would. I would have said yes to anything at that point.

A few days later, I got updated X-rays and started a weekly round of gel injections to help me survive my trip. Note that the word is "survive," not "thrive."

I did survive, but I had to opt out of so many activities and deal with such outrageous pain daily that, in hindsight, it was a poor decision to take that trip with the amount of pain I was experiencing.

At this point, my diagnosis had morphed from a minor recovery surgical procedure to a much more eye-popping diagnosis and recovery schedule.

After a thorough examination and studies of the X-rays and CT scans, both knees were diagnosed with "bone-on-bone" osteoarthritis, and the right knee appeared much worse than the left. This new diagnosis was not the news I wanted to hear.

I knew my knees were bothering me, and the pain was getting progressively worse, but I was surprised to find out I had bone-on-bone arthritis. I was active, took good care of myself, and maintained my weight.

It was hard for me to understand that osteoarthritis and human biology don't care about all that. In fact, human biology generally doesn't care how you *feel* about any of this.

I remember clearly the day I was given an option for a surgical procedure that would have been performed in an outpatient surgery center with about two weeks of recovery time. That surgical procedure could have helped reduce and possibly remove the daily pain I was experiencing in my right knee.

What did I say about that option? "TWO WEEKS of no travel? Are you kidding me? I have a BIG deal I'm working on. I can't possibly take time off right now, but I'll think about it after I close the deal. I'll find a better time. I promise."

Fast-forward 10 years ...

"Kicking the can down the road" led to the need for bilateral knee replacement—both knees at the same time. While this approach isn't commonly recommended, it was my choice.

Most people opt to replace their knees separately, spaced 3-12 months apart, to allow for better recovery and range of motion. In hindsight, I would advise others to take that staggered approach for the safest outcomes.

However, I was determined to pursue simultaneous replacement. I couldn't see myself undergoing two separate surgeries if there was a way to prepare for both at once. It wasn't a typical decision, but after negotiating with my medical team and carefully weighing the risks, I moved forward with replacing both knees together.

During my decade of "kicking the can down the road," I tried everything I could to deal with my knee pain. Overmedicating my pain with over-the-counter anti-inflammatory medicine and risking my kidneys and liver became a concern. Icing my joints and avoiding stairs were constants in my life.

Some of the things I tried to alleviate pain did work for a while—but then the fateful night came when I woke up in the middle of the night, heart pounding over a nightmare of being stabbed multiple times in the knees. The pain was now so extreme when I was sleeping that it was waking me up with nightmares.

That is when the incredible orthopedic surgeon I'm married to said, "You knee'd to know your time has come for surgery."

I'm thinking, *Why did this happen to me? I don't have time for surgery. I definitely don't have time for recovery.*

But there I was, in searing pain, knowing that if I didn't do something—and soon—I might end up in a wheelchair and addicted to painkillers. It happens to more people than you might think.

After my bilateral knee replacement surgery in October 2023, I learned firsthand the physical and mental toll this can take on somebody. I decided to document my experience online.

The American Academy of Orthopaedic Surgeons expects that by 2030, total knee replacements will grow to 3.5 million per year. About 60% of all knee replacement operations are performed on women. With those staggering figures, it became my mission to help others with their knee replacement adventure.

As a high-performance coach, patient, and lucky wife of an expert orthopedic joint replacement surgeon, it became my duty to help others undergoing joint replacement surgery.

My entrepreneurial journey started on the fourth day of my knee replacement recovery. While on painkillers and starting my recovery, I started building an app and website, thekneezone.com. My daily experiences became the framework for how to help others.

Sharing my post-op tips and mistakes to avoid led to coaching others through their knee replacements. Several people asked me to write a book, and during the writing process, my stepmother had knee replacement surgery. I was able to gift her with the first copy and get her real-time feedback on what worked and what was missing for her.

No Two Journeys Are the Same

It is crucial to remember that no two people are alike. We have different heights, weights, ages, medical histories, life experiences, and mindsets.

We are *not* all in the same boat.

We are in the same storm.

Some have yachts.

Some have canoes.

And some are drowning.

Some people will recover faster than others, some experience more pain than others, and some will tell you two weeks later that it was the best thing they ever did. Others may warn you not to do it.

Many people undergo replacement of both knees months or years apart. They are often surprised when the second knee replacement recovery is a different experience than the first, even with the same surgeon.

I can't predict your experience, but I can help give you a lifeboat as you enter the seas of this adventure.

If you want to learn from someone who has experienced knee replacements firsthand and has in-house expert advice from a surgeon on what to expect, how to prepare for, recover from, and even thrive after a knee replacement, you are in the right place.

> ### How Dr. Sinha Can Help
>
> As we write this book, I'm entering my 28th year as an orthopedic surgeon. For all 28 of those years, I have specialized in hip and knee arthroplasty, and I've performed over 10,000 hip and knee replacements.
>
> I also benefit from being involved in designing artificial knees and hips. Over a million patients worldwide currently have implants that I helped create. While those designs helped the vast majority of those people, I've also had the opportunity to witness some less-than-ideal designs by other surgeon teams, so I've learned what to avoid.
>
> In terms of patient care, I've also evolved from an era where we mainly focused on what surgeons thought was important to an era where we can tailor the operation so that patients can achieve what they're looking for in short-term and long-term recovery.
>
> I bring that vast experience and over 30 years of information-gathering to this book. Because of that, I can also provide generalities and specifics for individual patients and their particular situations.

Who This Book Is For

If you have been experiencing knee pain and want to learn more about avoiding, preparing for, recovering from, and thriving after a knee replacement, you are right where you need to be. We also wrote this book to help caregivers who will support another person on this "knee'd to know" adventure.

Caregivers are the unsung heroes of the recovery journey. If you are a caregiver reading this book, your dedication, patience, and encouragement will make a profound difference in the life of the person you support through knee replacement. Thank you in advance for being a source of strength and inspiration!

How to Read This Book

Depending on where you are in your "knee'd to know" journey, you may jump ahead to the chapter that will help you best right now in your journey. No worries. I'm good with that. We created this to allow readers to jump into the correct section that will help them when they get this book.

You may be early on in your journey and looking for ways to postpone surgery as long as possible. If so, skip to the end, where you'll learn "How to Avoid Surgery."

If you are preparing for surgery, read this book in order.

If you are a month into your recovery, skip to Weeks 2–4 of The Healing Journey.

Ask Dr. Sinha

People often ask me, "How do I know that I'm ready for surgery? I don't want to have surgery if I don't really need it. I also don't want to feel like I'm being a wimp and have the surgery too soon," to which I say, there are four things you should consider:

1. Nobody "needs" a knee replacement—knee replacement is for severe and debilitating pain from arthritis. Arthritis is not life-threatening, unlike heart disease or cancer. However, arthritis is *lifestyle* threatening, so you may eventually *want* a knee replacement to return to an active lifestyle.

2. Remember, the operation is primarily pain-relieving. And so, when your pain reaches the point where you start to avoid things that you would normally do because you know your knee is going to hurt afterward, when your friends and family members say to you, "Hey, you're not keeping up with us anymore," when you reach the point where you're sick and tired of being sick and tired, *that's* when you're ready to have surgery.

3. However, there is such a thing as waiting too long. So, if you let yourself become wheelchair-bound, knee replacement may not help you as much as you hoped. (This is discussed in more detail later in this book.)

4. Lastly, you must be physically and mentally committed to doing everything necessary to achieve a good outcome.

What We Hope This Book Will Provide for You

We created this book to empower you on your knee journey. Our mission is to share valuable insights from my personal experience—first postponing knee replacement, and then, when I finally took the exciting leap, preparing for and recovering from having both knees replaced at the same time.

We hope this uplifting journey, combined with expert advice from a knee replacement surgeon, will guide you toward recovery and renewed mobility.

I will also share stories of others with "bionic upgrades" whom I've coached through their rehabilitation. Everyone who undergoes a knee replacement has their own story to tell, and learning from others can be incredibly helpful. That said, I always caution against comparison during recovery. No two people are alike. Some will progress faster than others, but the ultimate goal is the same—to reach a point where you forget you even had your knee replaced.

Our overall goal is to help you understand what to expect, how to prepare, and how to navigate challenges so that, in time, you can not only recover but also *thrive* if you decide to replace your knee.

IS PUTTING IT OFF PUTTING YOU AT RISK?

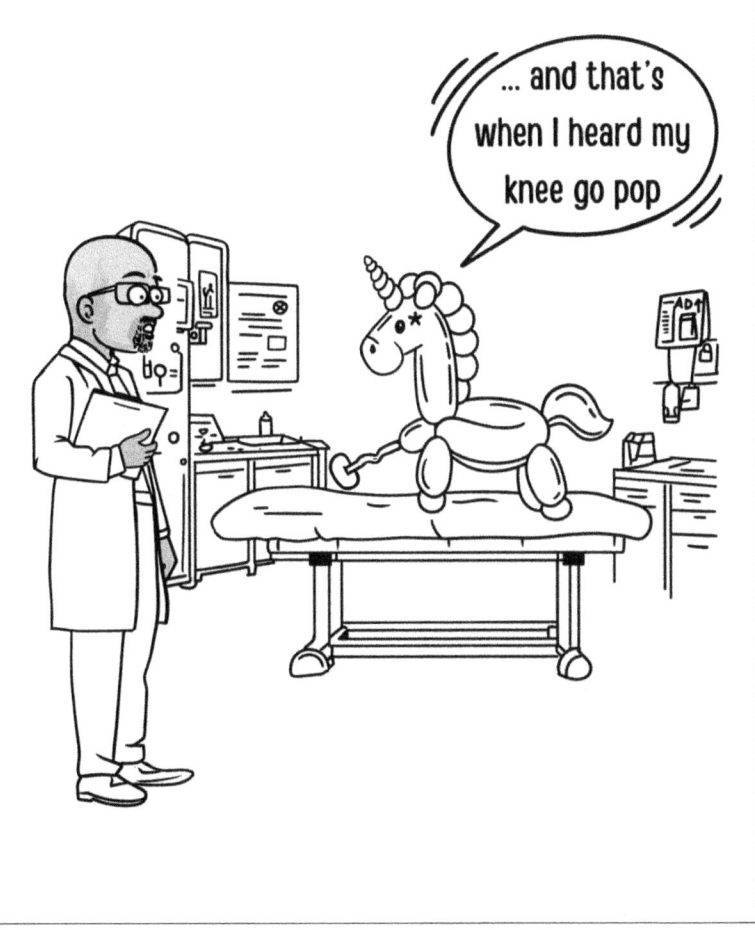

I'M TOO BUSY FOR SURGERY

How did I end up with bilateral knee replacement? I'm too stubborn for my own good, and I hope I have learned my lesson. My goal in sharing my story with you is that it might help if you face similar surgical options.

"Coulda, shoulda, woulda." How many times have we uttered that phrase? The beauty of life is that we get to reflect. At this point, it was ridiculous of me to think I shouldn't have taken time away from work to address the knee pain when several options were presented to me, including surgeries that would have been much simpler with less recovery time compared to total knee replacement.

One minor surgery would have been to operate only on my right knee, clean up a mess inside, and do a repair to provide better tracking of how the kneecap moved.

Another option along the way was a partial knee replacement.

These surgical options (suggested multiple times) would have required time off work, physical therapy, and certainly not wearing high heels for a while. I could not go to Pilates or play golf for a few weeks, and either option would have impacted my work-travel schedule.

When my surgeon presented these surgical options, I always had a big deal, big project, or big vacation planned, and making time to take care of myself would have interrupted them.

In hindsight, I should have taken the interruption. The other surgical options could have bought me much more time before needing a total knee replacement and *possibly* could have prevented knee replacement altogether. Instead, I was left with no other choice but total knee replacements. So, this chapter is for you go-getters, hustlers, and strivers!

I see you. I know you. I am you.

If you are advised to do a less invasive surgery earlier, please don't be stubborn and consider a few weeks' recovery versus a 6-12 month recovery from total knee replacement. Read that again, please—*weeks* as opposed to a year.

Because the less invasive surgery may provide you with:

1. A shorter recovery time: weeks vs. months
2. Less mental and physical impact on you than a total knee replacement
3. Ability to do some things easier, such as having a better range of motion (ability to bend your knee)

It is worth investigating whether it is better to spend a few weeks on the sidelines rather than months, usually up to a year, before fully recovering after total knee replacement. You could save time and money.

Maybe that less invasive option ship has sailed for you, or you're in the "I still want to keep trying options that don't include surgery" mindset. If this is you, jump over to the "How to Avoid Surgery" section at the end of the book and see all the things I tried to kick the can down the road until the painful nightmare hit me.

Dr. Sinha Weighs in on the Risks of Waiting Too Long

There is such a thing as waiting too long.

We get that information from our surgeon colleagues in Canada and England, where patients are on fairly long waiting lists for knee replacements. In America, the average time from deciding to have a knee replacement to having the surgery is approximately six weeks. In England and Canada, it can be 18 months or more.

We found that some patients in those countries have the means to get their surgery done elsewhere, like in the United States, and pay cash to have it done sooner. Those patients have better outcomes than their fellow citizens who have to wait 18 months.

The patients who had knee replacements sooner experienced less long-term pain, better early mobility, and better overall function.

We believe prolonged inactivity and lack of use due to pain cause muscle atrophy (loss of muscle fibers) and denervation (loss of nerve fibers). In some cases, even after the surgery, you never recover all of that lost muscle and nerve function.

That's why some patients have residual pain, stiffness, and weakness. Even though the operation was done well and the patient had done everything they could to recover correctly, because they waited too long, they never got to the point that they could have if they had been able to have the knee replacement surgery sooner.

Key Takeaways for Putting Off Surgery

1. Yes, there is such a thing as waiting too long for a knee replacement.
2. If you are experiencing knee pain, see a qualified orthopedic or sports medicine doctor for a proper diagnosis and understand your options.
3. The sooner you address the pain, the sooner you recover and thrive again.

WHAT YOU KNEE'D TO KNOW WHEN CONSIDERING TOTAL KNEE REPLACEMENT

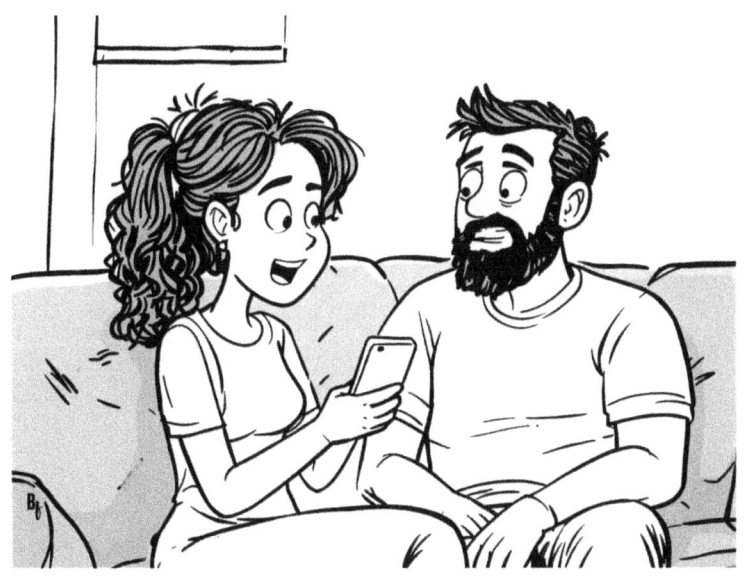

Can you believe it? I found information that the world's leading doctors don't know yet!

WHAT YOU "KNEE'D" TO KNOW BEFORE YOUR BIONIC UPGRADE

Having knee replacement—or what I like to call getting a "bionic upgrade"—is a big decision you should only make after considerable education. Knowing the essentials will help you decide if a bionic upgrade is right for you.

What is a total knee replacement? First and foremost, it is a major surgical operation. An orthopedic surgeon will remove the damaged ends of the bones of your knee joint and replace them with a metal and plastic artificial knee joint. For most people, it is less than an inch of bone. In fact, resurfacing of the joint is a more accurate description than replacement of the knee joint.

Before you embark on this journey, I will walk you through the 10 things you "knee'd" to know to prepare. As you proceed, I'll explore these big topics and explain what to expect in each recovery phase.

This surgery will require dedicated time on your behalf to recover. Below is a quick timeline of what to expect.

This list will help you with things to consider before the big bionic upgrade day. Think of it as an introduction to what you should learn before getting a knee replacement.

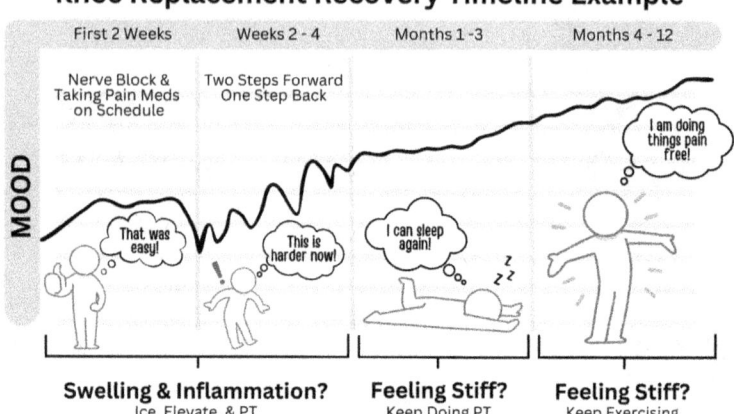

Who Should Consider a Total Knee Replacement?

An orthopedic surgeon is likely to recommend that you need a knee replacement if you experience the following:

- Severe pain that restricts work, walking, or daily and recreational activities
- Disturbed sleep due to night knee pain
- A very stiff knee that becomes swollen
- Advanced arthritis, as confirmed with X-rays
- Chronic pain that has not been relieved by the use of pain management, physical therapy, a cane, a walker, or resting
- Lack of blood supply (avascular necrosis), which has damaged the knee joint, usually caused by trauma/accident

Who Should *Not* Get a Total Knee Replacement?

Your orthopedic surgeon *may not* recommend a total knee replacement if you have any of the following:

- Severe obesity
- Severe peripheral artery disease
- Parkinson's disease
- Active infection
- Heart condition
- Lung disease
- Nerve disorder
- Metal allergy
- Poorly controlled diabetes
- Open wounds
- Severe edema
- Blood thinners

Every patient needs to be in optimal medical condition to limit surgical risks and improve chances of long-term success. People can have surgery with the above conditions under the right circumstances.

How Long Will My New Knee Replacement Last?

With the introduction of custom knee replacements and other technological advances, most people can expect the "bionic upgrade" to last 25-30 years. You can aid the lifetime of your knee replacement by maintaining a healthy weight and flexibility and avoiding strenuous impact sports that risk injury.

Near the end of this book, you'll find a comprehensive overview of the history of knee replacement, technology, and techniques, written by Dr. Sinha.

If you are still in the early stages of investigating your options for moving forward with a bionic upgrade, you may want to "jump" to that section now.

You'll gain a deeper knowledge of knee replacement, including:

- Quad-sparing surgical technique
- Robotic-assisted surgery
- The types of knee replacements available
- The importance of choosing the best surgeon

Look for "Dr. Sinha Comments on Technology and Modern Total Knee Replacement," which is just before our "Final Thoughts."

What Are the Top 10 Things I "Knee'd" to Know?

This surgery is a BIG decision and something that you should enter into with education before you begin. Here are my top 10 things you should know as you consider taking the next step, based on my personal experience and after helping coach others.

This list provides a quick summary of the significant items that should be on your research checklists:

1. Mindset
2. Choosing a surgeon
3. Insurance & co-pays

4. Home life
5. Sleep
6. Work impact
7. Driving
8. Travel & trips
9. Pain management
10. Physical therapy

In this section, I will share more about my journey, and you will hear from Dr. Sinha on what he also feels is most important from an expert knee replacement surgeon's experience.

Let's jump in—but don't hurt yourself.

The 10 Knee Replacement Essentials

1. Mindset

If we were sitting together, here is what I would ask you:

- Why do you want to get your knee replaced?
- What are the things you want to do that you can't do now with your knee pain?
- Do you avoid doing things you wish you could do?
- If we sit down this same time next year and you say, "I did it, and look at me now, I'm thriving," would that be enough motivation to help you through the tough days?
- Would you be willing to journal and keep a list of what you look forward to doing again?
- Are you mentally strong enough to push through the tough times after surgery in order to achieve your goals?

Why all these questions?

If you move forward on this journey, you will have at least one day when you wish you hadn't done this, and you will need to look at your list of "whys" to help keep you going.

If that list of "whys" doesn't have you jumping for joy about what you are excited about doing in your post-bionic upgraded life, we will need to sit longer and come up with the list that will have you jumping for joy.

You need a compelling "why" to get through this.

This surgery and recovery will require significant dedication, time, and patience on your part.

You can have the best surgeon and physical therapist in the world. Still, if you won't follow directions, make time for physical therapy, and understand that it will be months (up to 12, and in rare cases, up to 24) before you completely recover, you may want to rethink your "why."

Your attitude for every step of this journey will be vital in helping you get through this.

2. Choosing a Surgeon

You should research the best knee replacement surgeon in your area. You will not find this information on Yelp or Google.

So, how do you find the most skilled and lowest complications match for you?

Surgeon criteria checklist:

- ☑ Performs at least 100 knee replacements a year

- ☑ Fellowship trained
- ☑ Low complication rates

Since we know Dr. Google or Nurse ChatGPT will not give you the best answer, here are some suggestions:

- Go to medicare.gov to see a list of surgeon and hospital complication rates.
- Can you access physical therapists, operating room nurses, or orthopedic sales representatives in your area? If so, they will likely have recommendations on other patients' outcomes based on firsthand observations of orthopedic surgeons.
- Technical expertise is not the same as bedside manner. You want an expert surgeon. Let their staff be the friendliest, nicest people to you.
- Friends and family may have suggestions. If so, return to the first item on this list and research the surgeon once they make suggestions.

Once you find the best surgeon for you, you must share some vital information with the surgeon and staff.

Here is a list of things you should assemble to give you a head start:

- A list of your knee pain symptoms and what activities they are preventing you from doing
- What your long-term goals are
- Full medical and surgical history

- Allergies or poor reactions to anesthesia, adhesive surgical tapes, metals, and medications
- A complete list of ALL medications and supplements you take

If you think, suspect, or have sensitivities to adhesives or metals, it is imperative to share that with your doctor to ensure you are given the best options for your body. You don't want to risk infections or implant rejection. There are some options for people with metal sensitivities. Be sure to inform your surgeon if you suspect you have a metal sensitivity or known allergy.

3. Insurance, Medicare, & Co-Pays

It is essential to prepare in advance and understand your financial responsibility. If you are a US resident, this experience will likely involve receiving bills that your insurance may not cover.

Some people learn that co-pays for physical therapy can become quite expensive for several visits a week. The last thing you want to miss out on is your physical therapy after surgery.

Talk to your insurance company about your expenses in advance so you can budget and avoid surprises. Ask about options to discount out-of-pocket costs before they occur.

Here are some examples of items that might trigger bills or co-payments:

- Hospital/Surgery Center
- Orthopedic surgeon
- Anesthesiologist
- Physical therapy

- Equipment rentals: e.g., ice machine, ROMTech® Bike, continuous passive motion (CPM) machine
- Blood work
- Chest X-ray
- CT scan
- Knee X-ray

Your recovery rate will likely not improve as quickly when you receive shocking bills in the mail that you may not have expected.

Plan ahead with healthcare savings accounts (HSAs), deductibles, and the best insurance plan you can find.

4. Home Life Expectations

I coach people through what to expect at home immediately after knee surgery. Since everyone has different household responsibilities, planning can be invaluable.

Here are some high-level things I talk to people about to consider beforehand:

Cooking & Cleaning

I have both good news and bad news for you.

The good news? You won't be doing any cooking and cleaning.

The bad news? You won't be cooking and cleaning.

So, who will help?

You shouldn't be on your feet for long. Standing will cause swelling and discomfort. You'll need to assemble your care team *before* your big bionic upgrade day so you can focus on resting and recovering.

If you live alone, consider having prepared meals that are easy to reheat.

Can you stay with a family member or friend for a short period, or can they stay with you?

The Timer Game—Safely Returning to Activities

After about two to three weeks, I started "The Timer Game."

The game is played in 15-minute intervals. Set a timer or alarm on your phone to keep you from losing track of time.

Sit "toes above the nose" for 15 minutes. Then, stand for 15 minutes.

If that is going well and you have no increase in pain or swelling, you can increase your standing time by five-minute increments.

You must keep icing and elevating when you take that 15-minute sit break.

Think about only doing things that require little leg bending or turning.

Surgeons can tell when you haven't elevated and iced enough or, conversely, done too much activity. Your body is the perfect polygraph machine—it tells all.

Stairs

Using stairs immediately after your procedure can be very challenging. One option is to go sideways up the stairs, but if you can avoid stair-climbing for two to three weeks to regain some strength, do it!

We understand that you may have no choice. If that's the case, take it slow and steady and use a handrail. Going up, lead with your nonsurgical knee. Going down, lead with your surgical/bionic leg.

A quick way to remember is to lead *up* with the "good" and lead *down* with the "bad."

Need a visual demonstration? Check out the YouTube video link at:

TheKneeZone.com/education

Depending on how you came into the surgery with quadriceps strengthening, you might be okay with the stairs and regain your ability quickly. If you don't have good quad strength entering surgery, using the stairs will take longer to master.

Going downstairs confidently is usually one of the things that takes the longest to conquer after your knee replacement due to the amount of work required for quad strengthening.

Using stairs is much more challenging if you have a bilateral knee replacement. At five months, I could finally start going up and down flights of stairs properly without gripping the handrails for dear life.

I no longer fear stairs, but it took time, practice, and patience.

To build confidence *before* surgery, practice stepping up stairs with your (good) nonsurgical leg and stepping down with your (formerly bad) surgical leg. Remember, up with the good and down with the bad.

Help with Responsibilities

You will need a plan for at least the first week you are at home recovering from this major surgery. Other people at home may think they need your help (kids, spouse, parents), but during this time, you are the one who will need to be cared for. It's important to ask them (or others) for help.

Every day will get easier, but you need a plan on who will help cover your daily responsibilities and who will be available to help you. Equipment can also assist you with these activities, which we describe in more detail in the next chapter, "Preparing for Surgery."

Plan in advance who will help you with:

- Getting ice/ice packs
- Dressing and undressing
- Showering
- Taking medications on schedule
- Running errands if you need something

You should only need extra care for a week or two. Having additional help for the first two weeks will allow you to recover more quickly in the long run.

Pets, AKA Fur Babies

You might not like this next part if you are an animal lover and have a menagerie at home or even just one small pet you care for.

Just like humans, pets come in all shapes and sizes and require different things from you daily.

If you have a dog that requires walking, you will need to find someone else to take over that duty for a few weeks—it could be longer, depending on how well-behaved your dog is on a leash.

If you have a cat, place food and water bowls on a higher surface so you don't have to bend over as much. You should also consider doing the same with the litter box.

Your pets absolutely can't be near your operative knee. You can't risk an infection or injury to your incision. The last thing you want is an infection that can lead to terrible things.

Dr. Sinha once told me about a patient who had her dog lick her wound because she said, "Dog saliva has infection-fighting properties." It does—for the dog! Sadly, the patient got infected from the dog and had to have her knee replacement removed and replaced.

If your pets usually sleep with you, it's important to make other arrangements while you recover. As much as you may love their comfort and company, even a small movement or accidental bump can put your healing at risk. Keeping your sleep space safe gives your knee the best chance to recover fully. Protecting your sleep (and your new joint) is a top priority right now.

Please make sure you have a plan that allows you to recover safely with your pets.

Things you must prevent:

- Falling by tripping over your pet
- Your pet knocking you down by accident
- A pet jumping on your healing knee
- Your pet licking your wound once your bandage is off

If you have somebody at home to ensure your bird, rabbit, hamster, snake, cat, lizard, dog, or any other member of your menagerie can safely visit with you, you can spend quality time with your pets as long as you have safeguards in place. Pet gates can also be useful.

> ### Diana's Story: Fur Baby Precautions
>
>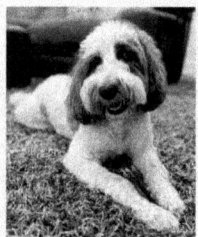
>
> *Here is Karma—this adorable Goldendoodle has more energy than you can imagine.*
>
> *Before my surgery, she had knocked me down several times by running behind me and jumping on me, thinking we were playing tag or some doggy chase game.*
>
> *When we scheduled my surgery, we knew we needed help with her. We got her extra training and an extended stay with friends and family until we could have several people at home with me to ensure Karma kept a safe distance until I was out of risk of getting an infection or injury.*

5. Sleep

If I could gift you sleep, I would. Sleeping can be very challenging for some people after surgery.

Helping people with sleep is one of the most significant services I provide in the early months of recovery. For some people, napping during the day makes falling asleep at night more difficult.

Ideally, you should sleep solo during the first week to protect your new knee.

Back Sleepers

- If you sleep on your back naturally, then you will likely get more sleep.
- Many people have found that it helps to sleep in a recliner for the first few weeks.
- Using a cervical pillow with a ridge that fits the curve of your neck will help prevent you from turning over and keep you on your back through the night.

Side Sleepers

- Sleeping on your side can be challenging and painful, although it is usually safe.
- After a few weeks, you can begin experimenting with sleeping on your side as your pain level decreases.
- To help you feel comfortable, you can put a squishy pillow, an airplane neck pillow, or a kid's plush toy under your knee or between your legs.

Stomach Sleepers

- It will be challenging and painful to sleep on your stomach, although it is safe to do so in most cases.
- After a few weeks, you can begin experimenting with sleeping on your stomach as your pain level and scar sensitivity decrease.

6. Work Impact

If you are still working or volunteering, you might wonder when you can return to work and how much time you need/get to take off.

When you can return to work is a difficult question to answer without knowing more about you and the demands of your job.

What do you do for work?

If you work remotely from home with a laptop, you will return to work quicker than somebody who climbs up and down a ladder for a living.

Your surgeon, physical therapist, and employer will help develop a plan based on the activity level your job requires.

- The average time off work, depending on your level of physical activity, is 6-12 weeks.
- Don't be in a big rush, as it will be more challenging than you think.
- Is a part-time return an option for you? Work-from-home?
- For ways to work at a desk and make your home recovery more comfortable, check out the "resources" section of thekneezone.com or scan the QR code below:

thekneezone.com/resources

7. Driving After Surgery

Your ability to return to driving will vary depending on which knee you have replaced.

You absolutely must be finished with prescription narcotics (painkillers) before you resume driving. The last thing you want is to be involved in an accident while healing.

- The average time for most people to return to driving is 3–6 weeks.
- No driving while taking narcotics.
- When you can safely drive again is something your surgeon will tell you based on your situation.
- The height of your vehicle is also essential. A high or low vehicle can leave you feeling humiliated or in pain.
- If you drive a manual transmission (stick shift), it may take longer to return to driving since it requires both legs and feet. It takes time to regain muscle strength and reflexes to have the proper strength to operate the clutch.
- You should be sure you can quickly move your foot from the gas to the brake pedal.
- If you plan to ride a motorcycle, you need an adequate range of motion, strength, and flexibility. Most people require 3–4 months before returning to motorcycle riding.
- Consider asking your surgeon about obtaining a temporary disability placard if you feel that would be helpful.

> ### Diana's Story: Getting Lifted Into an SUV
>
> *Once your surgeon clears you to drive, you may be "jumping" to enjoy a little getaway. Five months after my knee replacement, we took a trip.*
>
> *The rental car we ended up with was unexpectedly very low to the ground, so getting in and out of it was very challenging for me. On that same trip, our friends offered to drive us one night. They have an SUV lifted far off the ground with special shocks.*
>
> *I had to be lifted by two people to get into the SUV. I survived all these experiences, but I share them now so you can start thinking ahead.*

8. Travel & Trips

Returning to traveling takes an average of 4–6 weeks, depending on the type of trip, its length, and who will assist you.

Are business trips, family trips, or big dream vacations coming up?

Here is what to consider and how I help people prepare:

- How much walking is involved?
- Will there be steps or climbing involved?
- Are you carrying bags or rolling them very far, up and down ramps and stairs?
- Will you have access to ice and room to elevate your leg if needed?
- Will you be able to stand up and move around every two hours?
- Can you wear compression stockings to reduce swelling and reduce the risk of blood clots?

One concern about traveling in the first 6–12 weeks after surgery is the increased risk of blood clots, even on blood thinners.

When traveling on airplanes, the lower cabin pressure can cause swelling, which can lead to sluggish blood flow and clotting. Similarly, prolonged immobilization can do the same when traveling in the car for over an hour.

To ensure your safety, most surgeons recommend getting up every hour or so to walk and get your blood flowing.

9. Pain Management

Knee replacement is a very serious operation.

WARNING—GRAPHIC DESCRIPTION:

You are having your leg quickly cut off and reattached with that new bionic upgrade. We live in a wonderful time that offers replacement body parts!

You can hear everything that happens during a knee replacement and a detailed description of the surgery by going to:

thekneezone.com/education

- You will require medication on a strict schedule. Are you capable of taking medicine on an exact schedule to keep your pain under control?
- If you know you don't like certain pain relievers or have experienced allergic reactions to medications in the past, you must discuss this with your surgeon.
- The biggest thing I hear causing problems the first few weeks is people not following the pain management schedule and then being in horrible pain.
- You must stay ahead of the pain by keeping on a schedule.

10. Physical Therapy

You will need to be on a physical therapy program to experience a full recovery.

- You may have the option to have physical therapy at home, at a facility, or even via video or an app on your phone.
- Your insurance might cover access to an exercise bike. I used a ROMTech bike, which I credit for helping me recover quickly.
- You must learn and practice exercises daily for the first few months.
- This surgery is akin to running a marathon, not a sprint. You must be consistent with your daily physical therapy training homework to have a successful recovery.
- You will also need to massage your knee and leg to break up scar tissue that will rapidly form.

> ### Dr. Sinha Comments on What to Expect from Having Knee Replacement Surgery
>
> For patients with advanced knee arthritis who have started down some treatment path and are starting to get close to surgery, the common question is, "Well, what does surgery involve? What am I going to go through?"
>
> I tell them the following: the surgery takes about an hour to an hour and a half. About half the patients go home the same day. If a hospital stay is required, it is typically one night. In 99.9% of cases, you'll be allowed to put full weight on the replaced knee immediately. In fact, you'll be up walking on the day of surgery.

I typically have everybody start using a walker for about two weeks because you have to get used to this new leg, and I want to protect the surgical wound. I don't want you to stumble or fall and cause the wound to come open.

After two weeks, if you feel comfortable enough to move to a cane, we'll have you do that. You don't have to switch to a cane after two weeks. If you still feel like you need the walker, *that's okay.*

You're probably ready to start driving once you're comfortable walking with a cane. The data suggests that it takes about six weeks to get your reaction time back after surgery to drive as well as you did before. I agree with that.

However, I've found that once people have enough leg control to walk with a cane, they have enough leg control to get in and out of a car safely and move their foot from the gas to the brake safely. But if you're still taking a lot of narcotic pain medications, it's not safe (for you and other drivers!) to be out on the road.

Physical therapy lasts about 4–12 weeks, depending on where you started initially and if your insurance will allow it. In my practice, we initially set up physical therapy at home, where the therapist comes to your house for the first two to three weeks.

Afterward, we'll transition you to outpatient therapy, where you go to a physical therapy office. The physical therapy office has a lot more equipment to help with pain reduction, swelling reduction, muscle strengthening, walking, and balancing. For optimal recovery, try to do the exercises from physical therapy at home every day if you can.

Key Takeaways for Considering a Total Knee Replacement

These are the most important questions to help you decide whether it is time for a bionic upgrade.

1. Are you missing out on too many things you want to be doing without pain?
2. Is your pain past the point of no return daily—remember my stabbing nightmares?
3. Are you mentally ready? Do you have your list of "WHYS" to help you get through the bad days?
4. Can you commit to learning and completing your daily physical therapy exercises? This answer MUST be a YES if you want a successful outcome.

> **Are You Still With Me?**
>
> *If you feel confident you can manage all these things, you're ready to move forward. I want to help you prepare for your total knee replacement.*
>
> *Onward we go—let's leap to pre-hab together.*

PREPARING FOR SURGERY

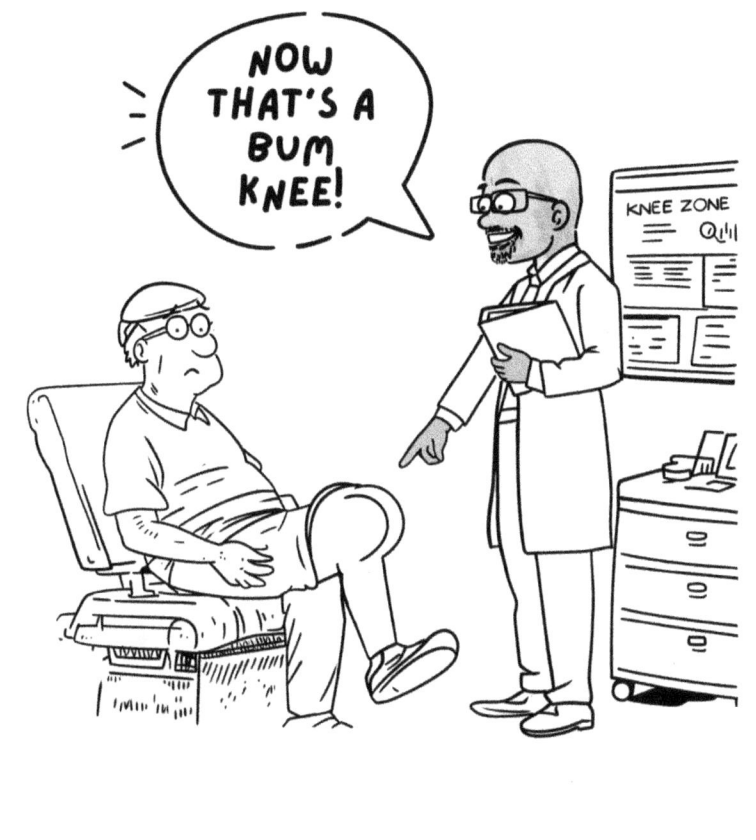

PRE-HAB FOR KNEE REPLACEMENT

Once I decided to replace both my knees simultaneously, my focus shifted. I was curious about how to prepare myself for the best experience. This decision was a significant mind shift after a decade of denial. I suddenly craved information on the best way to get ready.

You play a significant role in your recovery after surgery by performing physical therapy exercises daily. Starting some exercises before your surgery will help you get into a rhythm that will support you after surgery as well.

Admittedly, I had a massive advantage in marrying an expert joint replacement surgeon. I started asking him lots of questions about what I could do to ensure I entered into surgery as physically prepared as possible.

When I first heard somebody using the phrase "pre-hab," I was at a Pilates class, cringing in pain with every squat I attempted. I shared with the instructor, Megan, that I was going to have my knees replaced.

Megan enthusiastically said, "Great, Diana, you should do as much pre-hab as possible to prepare." The concept of pre-hab, or pre-rehabilitation, stuck with me.

You must prepare to set yourself up for success during the recovery phase. Like people training for a marathon, you must prepare for a great outcome before the day of the marathon.

I knew that I would need to be prepared both physically and mentally if I was going to be able to have both knees replaced. Again, having both knees replaced simultaneously is not recommended in many circumstances.

Here's What I Did to Get Ready:

Physical Preparation Pre-Hab

If possible, go to physical therapy before your surgery. If that isn't an option, you can watch YouTube videos online or your insurance may offer something online.

- Quads, quads, quads—you can't over-strengthen your quads while getting ready for this surgery. During your knee replacement surgery, your quadriceps tendon, which is attached to your quadriceps muscle, gets cut and then stitched back together. That small cut will weaken the tendon and muscle as a result. It will typically take three months for the tissue to heal. By strengthening your quads before surgery, you will have some strength remaining after your surgery. My YouTube channel, The Knee Zone, has free examples of what to do.
- You can also buy online classes. Physical therapist Dr. Samantha Smith runs an online forum for knee patients. Check out our website for a complete list of resources to help you get what you need for your knee replacement or scan the following QR code:

thekneezone.com/resources

- Upper body strengthening—you will use those arms more than you realize for the first two to three weeks to help you get up.
- Learn to use a walker, crutches, or cane ahead of surgery.

Surgery Preparation

Going into surgery, I wanted to be in the best physical shape possible. That meant reviewing my eating and drinking habits, which your surgeon will also recommend.

- I decided 90 days before surgery to be alcohol-free. I wanted to be clear-minded and free of as much inflammation as possible.
- I stayed focused on losing unwanted weight and keeping a healthy BMI.
- I don't smoke, but if I did, you can bet I would have stopped that as well.
- Do your best to have a bowel movement the night before your surgery, or be as "regular" as possible the day before.

Other Important Precautions

- **Sleep.** Try to get a full night of sleep before surgery so you're well-rested.
- **Dental work.** Get your cleanings and any other dental work done before surgery. You want to avoid an infection after surgery, and dental work can increase your risk of infection.
- **Stay healthy.** The last thing you want is to become sick before surgery. If you need to be around a bunch of people right before your surgery, "mask up" so you don't risk canceling your bionic upgrade.
- **Cigarettes.** Best to quit smoking six or more weeks ahead of surgery. Very serious and life-threatening complications can occur, including pneumonia, stroke, heart attack, constricted blood circulation, and impaired wound and bone healing.
- **Heavy drinkers, beware.** People who drink heavily (three drinks per night) run the risk of their body going into withdrawal if they quit drinking suddenly. If you are a heavy drinker, discuss a plan to decrease your consumption slowly and not risk withdrawal and your life.
- **Marijuana, THC, illicit drugs.** Recreational drugs are particularly problematic around surgery and anesthesia because of the negative interactions they will have with commonly used medications. Don't partake for at least 72 hours before your surgery.
- **Increase your protein intake.** Many people enter surgery malnourished. Your protein needs before and after knee replacement surgery increase to maintain muscle mass, support bone health, enhance immune function, and promote healing.

Diana's Story: My Last Blast Before Surgery

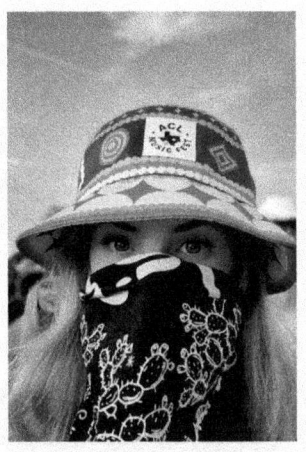

I wanted to see Alanis Morissette, Shania Twain, Mumford & Sons, Foo Fighters, Noah Kahan—and, well, the list was long—so I figured this would be my last blast before my bionic upgrades to enjoy the fun with friends.

My approach to attending the Austin City Limits (ACL) Music Festival was different from years past. The year before my surgery, I chose to:

- *Mask up and wear a bandana over it to help protect myself from dust and picking up an unwanted bug.*
- *Stay behind the crowds and sit on blankets for most performances.*
- *Give myself lots of extra time to walk, as this venue required plenty of walking.*
- *Take over-the-counter (OTC) medications on a rigorous schedule to deal with the pain.*
- *Stay hydrated with as much water as I could handle.*

All in all, I had fun, but it was exhausting. I only made it through two of the three nights of the event.

Home Prep

You will need to plan for the surgery by getting some things in your house ready to make it easier once you return home from surgery.

- **Stairs.** To get in and out of the house, do you need to use the stairs? Are there stairs inside? If you must use stairs at home, ensure you learn how to use them before leaving the hospital.
- **Meals.** Plan each of your meals for the first week home.
- **Entertainment.** Keep your mind occupied with books, magazines, TV series, journaling, etc. Ensure you have the power cords nearby and maybe replace the batteries in the remotes ahead of time.
- **Sleep.** Can you sleep solo for the first few days to avoid having your knee bumped? Also, if you usually sleep on your side, it can be challenging. Ensure your bed is not too low or too high to the ground.
- **Nightlights.** They help with visibility for when you get out of bed. They also help with any disorientation you might experience during the night, sometimes caused by the pain medications.
- **Rugs.** Pick up any throw rugs that you could trip on.
- **Furniture.** Look at the height of the furniture in your home.
    - If your favorite chair:
        - Requires a deep knee bend to sit down, you will find it extremely difficult to stand up later.
        - Has wheels, then it is dangerous and you shouldn't use it.

- Doesn't have arms on it to push off from, it will be hard to get up.
  o If your sofa is too low to sit on comfortably, you can try a few things:
    - Stack cushions to raise the seat height.
    - Pile some pillows to raise the seat height.
    - Place a block of wood or bricks under the legs.
  o Practice sitting on the chair and sofa, and push yourself forward to the edge to stand up if the seat depth is an issue.
- **Toilet.** The height of the toilet is very important.
  o Practice to see if you can sit down and get up using one leg.
  o Don't use a toilet paper holder for support—it will come off the wall.
  o For toilet-support options, check out the "resources" section of thekneezone.com or scan the QR code below:

thekneezone.com/resources

- **Comfort.** Plan in advance where you will spend most of your time the first week—your perfect place to ice and elevate.
  - Find a chair with armrests high enough that your knees don't have to bend past 90 degrees when you sit. The chair arms allow you to use your arms to lower yourself down and push yourself up.
  - To elevate your surgical leg, find something you can move in front of the chair and pile on pillows to achieve the proper elevation.
  - Remember, toes ideally are higher than your nose, and nothing is ever under the knee.
  - Equipment that will make your first few weeks easier: toilet riser, walker, and car cane. Find links to these and more on our website or scan the QR code below:

thekneezone.com/resources

Work Impact

- Let people know you are having *major* surgery as soon as possible so everybody can plan how they are going to survive without you.

- Find out what paperwork your company's disability insurance carrier will need from your surgeon for your medical leave, and do so well in advance.
- Ensure you have the email addresses and phone numbers of people you need to contact written down and available in case you rely on your work computer for everything and are locked out of it while on medical leave.
- Your time off to recover will vary depending on your work—sitting, standing, or strenuous labor—and based on your surgeon's suggestion and medical needs.

Driving After Surgery

- No driving on narcotics!
- You won't be able to drive right away. Plan ahead for someone who can help you with transportation if you need to see your surgeon or go to physical therapy.
- The average time before driving is three weeks if your left knee is replaced and six weeks if your right knee is replaced.
- If you drive a manual transmission and have had your left knee replaced, you must ensure your leg is strong enough to operate the clutch. This process takes 4–6 weeks on average.
- The height of your vehicle is also essential to consider. Being too high or too low can be challenging and impact your ability to drive safely.

Dental Work

- If you need any dental work or cleaning, do it before your surgery.
- To protect yourself against infections, you will have restrictions for the first six weeks immediately after your surgery, such as not seeing a dentist for nonemergency work.

Childcare or Others You Care For

- YOU are the one who will need care.
- Ensure everybody knows you cannot help until you feel ready.
- You cannot easily get down on the floor and back up. This lack of mobility also makes picking up a child nearly impossible. You don't want to risk injuring a child or yourself.

Pet Care

- If you have pets, who will care for them after your surgery?
- Pets are a great comfort but can also increase the risk of falling or infecting your new knee.

Communication Plan

- Your adoring friends and family will want updates on how you are doing. You will be exhausted and may not have the energy to respond to every text and message you get.

- Using a platform like Caring Bridge makes inviting people to hear about your updates easy. One post and everybody knows how you're doing.
- Be proactive and ask a friend or family member to let everyone know how you're doing on your behalf.
- Consider creating a special group text you'll use for the first 48 hours.

Hospital Packing List

If you know you are spending the night, the following might be helpful:

- Earplugs
- Eye mask
- Reading material
- Phone/tablet charger and extension cord
- Glasses (contacts are not a good idea at the hospital)
- Loose-fitting clothing: sweatshirt or sweater, pants or shorts
- Toothbrush, toothpaste, and lotion
- Easy shoes to wear home—do not bring flip-flops! Your feet might be swollen.

Put them all in a bag with your name on it so it is easy to keep track of them.

About Alcohol & Marijuana/THC

Drinking alcohol or using anything with THC before surgery can increase the risk of complications during and after the procedure. These complications could affect:

- **Anesthesia.** Alcohol & THC can interfere with anesthesia, which may require higher doses during surgery.
- **Medications.** Alcohol & THC can also interfere with other medications, causing them to work differently, especially blood thinners.
- **Wound healing.** Alcohol & THC can delay wound healing.
- **Infections.** Alcohol & THC can increase the risk of surgical site infections.
- **Bleeding.** Alcohol & THC can increase bleeding episodes during surgery.
- **Heart and lung problems.** Alcohol & smoking marijuana can lead to pulmonary complications that affect the respiratory system.
- **Recovery time.** Alcohol & THC use can increase surgical recovery time.

Some surgeons recommend avoiding alcohol for at least two weeks before surgery, while others suggest cutting it out longer. Marijuana and THC products should be stopped a minimum of 72 hours before surgery.

Must-Haves, Nice-to-Haves, and Prescribed Specialty Items

Things you absolutely must have:

- **Ice packs.** You need flexible gel ice packs. Have plenty on hand if you don't get an ice machine.
- **Walker.** You will likely be leaving the hospital with one (it's often provided to you directly).
- **Toilet riser.** Depending on your height, you may want this to raise the toilet seat to make it easier to get on and off.
- **Shower chair.** A plastic chair for your shower with non-slip feet and no wheels.
- **Three-in-one shower chair.** This portable bedside commode doubles as an elevated seat over the toilet and then triples as a shower chair.
- **Bell.** (LOL) In all seriousness, you will want a way to alert people to help you when you need help in the first few days. Have something you know will get their attention—a bullhorn, cowbell, yelling for help, whatever it takes.

Are there other things you might want that would be nice to have?

- **Ice machine.** Using an ice machine helps reduce your pain and swelling.
- **Grabber.** A grabber can help you pick up things that are just out of reach.

- **Leg-lifter strap.** A leg-lifter strap will help you move your leg and can help with physical therapy exercises.
- **Shower sleeve.** A shower sleeve is handy for covering your leg in the shower the first few times to protect your bandage if it isn't waterproof.
- **Mini skateboard.** A mini skateboard can assist with range-of-motion exercises.
- **Stationary bicycle or peddler.** A stationary bike was one of the most valuable things I used during my recovery. Peddling can help speed up the healing process.
- **TENS unit.** Electric stimulation from a TENS unit is helpful for quad activation, muscle relaxation, and pain management.
- **The Kneely Pad.** Use a knee pad like The Kneely Pad to assist you with kneeling once your surgeon allows you to begin kneeling.
- **Car Cane.** This is an ergonomic car handle that will allow you to get in and out of the car without fear of falling.

Specialty items that your surgeon might prescribe:

- **Game Ready® Ice Machine** for compression and cold therapy.
- **ROMTech PortableConnect** for gentle therapeutic movement to increase range of motion and speed healing.
- **Continuous Passive Motion (CPM)** machine to reduce joint stiffness and increase range of motion.

You can find links to some of our specialty item recommendations by scanning the QR code below or going to the "resources" section of thekneezone.com:

thekneezone.com/resources

Mindset

I kept a journal of everything I looked forward to doing once I recovered. This list of things you are excited about will help you stay motivated during the recovery phases!

READ what your surgeon's office gives you in advance. It will contain the necessary instructions to follow to be ready for your surgery.

What Dr. Sinha Says About Getting Ready for Your Surgery

The concept of pre-rehabilitation, or pre-hab, is not new. We first started talking about it in the late 1990s, and in fact, the first research paper I wrote about the importance of muscle strength around joint replacement surgery was in 1999.

The basic idea is that if you're stronger going into the operation, you'll be stronger coming out of it. If you think about it this way, this makes the most sense. When you stop using your knee because it hurts from arthritis, the muscles around the joint aren't used either. And if the muscles aren't used, they lose their muscle tone, size, and overall strength.

It's like the age-old saying: if you don't use it, you lose it. Well, that's very true in this situation. In addition, when we perform the operation, we traumatize the muscles, which makes them even weaker than before the surgery. Whenever you have surgery, there is some swelling that causes muscles not to contract.

In your overall recovery, you must overcome all the things that cause your muscles to weaken. If you pre-rehabilitate your muscles before going into surgery, you'll start from a higher standpoint of muscle function, and you won't see as much decrease in muscle function in the early recovery phase. It will allow you to recover faster if you can rehabilitate your quadriceps muscles and become stronger going into the operation.

Key Takeaways for Preparing for Surgery

1. If you have time before surgery, do some pre-hab to help you prepare.
2. Mindset is a key focus when it comes to helping you stay positive and having others assist you.
3. I can't emphasize this enough: **READ** what your surgeon's office gives you before your surgery and *follow the instructions.*

THE BIG BIONIC UPGRADE DAY

It's 5 a.m., and it's dark outside. You are at the hospital, sitting in the waiting room. You have a fancy new wristband and have signed your name more times in 15 minutes than you can count.

All of a sudden, you feel scared, nervous, and angry. That gnawing memory of "Why me?" has crept back into your mind, stomping its foot like an angry toddler.

You feel your heartbeat accelerating and wonder, "Is this going to be ok?"

Take a deep breath in for four counts. Hold it for a second and a half. Let it out for eight counts.

You are ready!

Take another deep breath in. Hold it. Let it out.

You have trained for this.

Deep breath in. Deep breath out.

You are prepared!

Keep breathing!

What to Expect on Your Bionic Upgrade Day

Your surgeon's office will provide you with a guide on preoperative instructions. *Please read and follow these instructions.*

Depending on your surgeon's plans, your overall health, and your type of insurance, you may spend a night in the hospital or be in a surgery center for the day.

While you're waiting to be called into surgery, you might want to go over your post-op plan or review your "why" with the support person who came with you.

When you hear them call your name, take another deep breath, kiss and hug the person sitting with you, and hand them your phone and personal items. You will see them soon after the surgery is over.

A nurse will escort you to an area to change into your surgical outfit and store your clothing. Your surgical outfit will consist of a hair bonnet, gown, and grip socks, so you'll be ready for that first walk in a few hours.

You will likely have a friendly nurse to take your vitals and prepare you for an IV.

Your surgeon will meet with you. They will autograph your surgical leg so you both agree this is the knee you are having replaced. If you have both knees replaced, you will discuss which knee they will replace first.

Then, an anesthesiologist will visit. I nicknamed mine "Dr. Candy Man" and told him I would like a generous dose of the "I don't want to remember being here" version of whatever he had planned to give me.

Lucky for me, he found that request amusing. The anesthesiologist will ask you a few more questions about your history with anesthesia. If you have had any issues with anesthesia, please let them know so they can consider using other options to ensure you have the best experience.

Things move pretty quickly from here. In my case, they rolled me into the operating room, where my friendly nurse, anesthesiologist, and surgeon were ready. You may feel the operating room is cold. This is normal. The room needs to be a certain temperature to reduce the risk of infection and ensure your hard-working surgeon and surgical team are comfortable once they are in there.

Next, the nurse asked me to sit up, rotate to the edge, dangle my legs over the side of my rolling bed, and hold a pillow to my stomach to receive the spinal block. That is the last thing I remember until I woke up in recovery after the surgery.

Dr. Candy Man did an excellent job meeting my request: "I don't want to remember or feel anything."

> *If you want to see what happens during the surgery or hear a great description of what happens, you can find viewing options on the education page at thekneezone.com.*

Recovery Room—*Congratulations!*—You Are Now Bionic!

When you awake from anesthesia, you may feel great, tired, nauseous, giggly, or confused. You may also feel thirsty and hungry. Be sure to share how you feel with the recovery room nurse so they can help you feel better.

Once the nursing team feels you are comfortable and alert, they will let your family or friends know they can come and sit with you and bring your personal belongings. You will still be in your surgical outfit—minus the hair bonnet.

You may have compression stockings on your legs.

Spoiler Alert: In the coming days, you will likely wish you had the hair bonnet back instead of the compression stockings.

The recovery room nursing teams will closely monitor your pain levels.

- You absolutely **must** stay ahead of the pain.
- Be vocal if you are uncomfortable—tell someone ASAP!
- The good news is that you will likely not feel any discomfort.
- That nerve block works so well that you might even think this was a complete piece of cake. *What was I so worried about when I got here this morning?*

PRO TIP: This is not the time to be a hero.

A physical therapist or recovery room nurse from the hospital or surgery center will come to see you next. This is the exciting part … You will be up and walking around the same day as your surgery!

The physical therapist will teach you how to use the walker and ensure you can safely stand up and take those exciting first steps. This phase is amazing! Here you are, up and walking on that NEW KNEE.

Your surgeon and physical therapist will have a plan of what you must accomplish before you leave the hospital or surgery center.

Stairs

If you must climb stairs in your home, tell the physical therapist so you can practice before you go home. You must lead with your nonsurgical leg and step down using your surgical leg when climbing stairs. You will be taught by a physical therapist how to use the stairs before you leave to return home.

Restroom Requirements

You will likely be required to use the restroom safely on your own after the surgery and before you can be discharged from the hospital. You will also be expected to urinate and possibly have a bowel movement before leaving. Performing these actions is essential because it indicates that your bodily systems function correctly.

Many people suffer constipation as a side effect of anesthesia, pain medication, and dehydration. If you find you're not having bowel movements on your normal schedule, be aggressive using laxatives—not just stool softeners—because constipation may cause your pain medications to be less effective.

During the surgery, you may be given a urinary catheter device. A catheter may leave a lingering effect once you return home. Be sure to monitor yourself for any signs of a urinary tract infection and get antibiotics immediately from your surgeon. You don't want an infection of any kind after your surgery.

Time to Go Home

Your surgeon or physician's assistant (PA) will come by to see you. After they examine what they removed during the surgery, they will tell you how much you truly needed that bionic upgrade you just received.

You will eventually get ready to go home. You might go home the same day or the next day. Depending on your overall health, your surgeon may keep you in the hospital. A night in the hospital is nothing to worry about. Your surgeon wants to ensure the best outcome for you.

In my case, I was allowed to leave the hospital on the second day. Bilateral knee replacements are not as common, and since recovery is much more challenging, staying in the hospital to control pain, monitor swelling, and master walking on two new knees takes more time.

You should change your clothes before going home. Wear something easy to put on, such as loose shorts. You might need help with underpants and socks. That nerve block makes it hard to move, and your swollen knee will restrict movement. You might find yourself needing to use your arms to move your leg. Don't panic if moving your leg is nearly impossible without manually lifting it.

When you get ready to leave, double-check that you have everything you need: phone, charging cables, glasses, the clothes you wore when you arrived, books, etc.

You may feel some "brain fog," so take your time and double-check.

Say goodbye and thank all the friendly people who cared for you.

You will get to ride in a wheelchair out to your vehicle.

This is where you show off how well you listened to your physical therapist about standing up and using the walker.

Getting Into the Car

1. Be sure the vehicle's height is manageable—getting into a lifted truck or a low sports car will be really difficult.
2. Position the front passenger seat as far back as possible.
3. Put the window down and open the door as wide as you can.

4. Approach the passenger seat with your back facing the seat by carefully using your walker.
5. Back up gently until you feel the car right behind you.
6. Let the driver take your walker away while you hold the car door.
7. Keep your bionic leg a step forward and hold on to the windowsill and car frame for support.
8. Slowly bend your head and chest forward, sticking your bottom out until it makes contact with the seat. Sigh with relief.
9. Watch your head and slide onto the seat securely.
10. Slowly turn toward the front of the car and lift one leg in after the other. At first, you may need to help lift your bionic leg into the car.
11. Sit forward, exhale, and remind yourself that this will get easier each time. Then, close the door, and off you go.

Bonus Tips for the Car

- Leather can stick to your skin in warm weather. If you stick to the seat and it is hard to turn, you can put a plastic garbage bag or towel on the seat to help you turn more easily.
- If you are tall and stretching your bionic leg is difficult, you can sit sideways on a bench seat in the back until you improve your range of motion.
- An ergonomic car handle called a "car cane" allows you to get in and out of the car without fear of falling. You can find links to some of our specialty item

recommendations by scanning the QR code below or going to the "resources" section of thekneezone.com:

thekneezone.com/resources

> ### Dr. Sinha's Experience
>
> You will come in on the day of surgery and get checked in. The nurse will start IV(s), dress you with foot pumps and compression socks, and go through a bunch of paperwork.
>
> You'll meet with the anesthesiologist, who will talk to you about what type of anesthetic they're going to use. I prefer a combination of four things for anesthesia. I'll talk about that below.
>
> Once the anesthetic is decided upon, you'll go to the operating room. You'll either be given a spinal or a general anesthetic as the primary method. Either way, you'll be given heavy sedation, so you won't remember anything that's going on.
>
> The surgery will happen, and when it's done, you'll wake up in the recovery room.
>
> There are two different types of anesthesia commonly used for knee replacement.

One is called general anesthesia. That's where a breathing tube is placed into your mouth and throat, and a machine breathes for you during the operation.

The second is called spinal anesthesia. That's where the anesthesiologist puts a needle into your back around your spine, *not into your spine*, and they inject an anesthetic that numbs you from the waist down.

The most significant advantage of the spinal is that you breathe on your own, so when the spinal anesthetic wears off, you don't have that feeling of being hit by a truck as you do with general anesthesia.

When they put you deep under using general anesthesia, they have to use very heavy sedation and muscle paralyzers, which have to be reversed for you to wake up fully. Sedation with spinal anesthesia is not as deep and is short-acting.

There are specific reasons to use both types, such as previous back surgery or certain heart conditions. Your anesthesiologist and surgeon should discuss the pros and cons of each as they pertain to you specifically.

I also like to use a nerve block ahead of time. The major sensory nerves in your knee reside in an area called the adductor canal. So we do an adductor canal block that numbs the front of the leg for about six hours.

Then, in surgery, I'll inject a pain management cocktail that has anesthetics, anti-inflammatory medicines, and epinephrine all around the tissues. This injection helps the adductor canal nerve block last longer and numbs the back of the knee.

The last thing I do is coat the tissues with a slow-dissolving combination of meloxicam (anti-inflammatory) and bupivacaine (anesthetic). That doesn't get rid of all your pain, but it blocks about 70–80% after the surgery. As a result, you need less narcotic medication, which is a good thing.

Once you've completed the recovery room period, which typically lasts 45 minutes to an hour, you'll go to your room. A little later, the physical therapist will come by and teach you some exercises.

No matter what type of anesthesia you had, you should be awake and feeling minimal pain thanks to the nerve blocks. This allows you to get out of bed and walk around your room. However, when the nerve blocks wear off, if you're not prepared, the pain can hit suddenly and hard, making you feel like you fell off a cliff.

Before that happens, we start to preload you with medications. In fact, it starts before the surgery. We begin to give you medications in the preoperative area to help block pain after the surgery.

During the first day or so in the hospital, we'll give you certain medications on a regular schedule, even if your pain is zero. If your pain gets above that, though, there's a whole sliding scale of how strong of a pain medication to get. You just have to ask for it.

The goal is to keep your pain below "3" out of "10" in the first 24 hours. The reason is that the data shows that if you control your pain in the first 72 hours really well, you wind up using less pain medication overall in your recovery than if you let your pain get out of control.

In addition, most modern protocols try to reduce opioid consumption in total by using an approach called multi-modal pain management. In this technique, multiple medications such as anti-inflammatories, tramadol, gabapentin, and acetaminophen are used in smaller dosages to limit the need for opioids.

Within the past decade or so, at least in the United States, there has been a movement toward same-day discharge after knee replacement. Whether you have the surgery in a hospital or an ambulatory surgery center (commonly called an ASC), you must meet specific criteria to go home the same day. In patients who meet the criteria, same-day discharge is safe and has been shown not to have higher complication rates.

Key Takeaways for Your BIG Bionic Upgrade Day

1. Long, slow, deep breaths will help you stay calm if anxiety creeps in at any point.
2. Communicate honestly with the staff about how you are feeling.
3. Keep track of the names of the people helping you and thank them by name. You can also name them on the survey you will likely receive from the hospital later.
4. Add a basket or tote bag to your walker to easily transport things around.

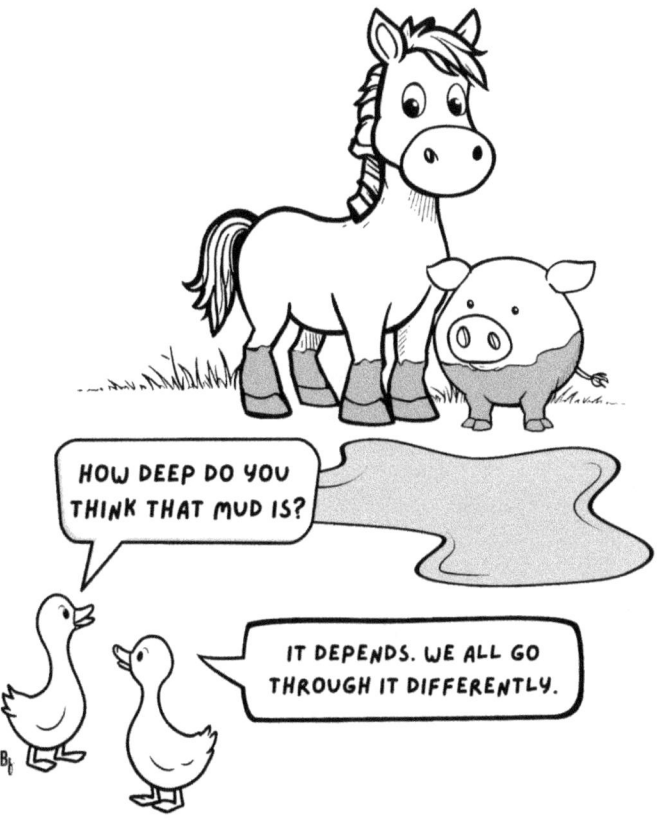

WEEKLY RECOVERY GUIDE
WEEKS 1 & 2

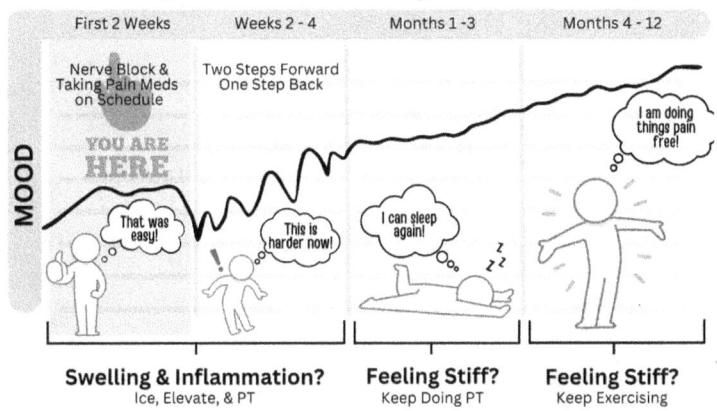

Once you are home from the hospital, you will likely have that nerve block still working, preventing pain, and you might be thinking this surgery wasn't hard or painful at all.

Why was Diana so emphatic about telling me to be prepared?

You will be fine, my friend. However, that nerve block will wear off soon, and things are about to change.

You will be feeling "all the feels."

Weeks 1 & 2 require you and whomever you have to help you stay on schedule.

Staying on your schedule is the only way to avoid a setback and recover successfully.

Here are the critical things for Weeks 1 & 2 and how to help manage them.

1. Pain Medication Schedule
2. Sleep
3. Stairs
4. Potty Talk
5. Showering Tips
6. Physical Therapy/Exercises
7. RICE—Rest, Ice, Compression, Elevate
8. What to Do With Your Newfound Time
9. Have a Schedule—And Stick With It
10. Low Furniture
11. Skin Irritation and Reactions
12. Leaving the House
13. Mental Health Check-In

Pain Medication Schedule

You will be prescribed a variety of prescription medications to take on a schedule after your surgery.

YES, you need to take them. Your surgeon has given you pain medication to help you "stay ahead of the pain."

Once the nerve block has worn off, you will suddenly feel pain. To keep it to a minimum, it is crucial to follow the surgeon's schedule.

You can find an easy pain medication template by going to the "resources" section of our website, thekneezone.com, or by scanning the following QR code:

TheKneeZone.com/resources

Are you feeling nauseated or having severe brain fog from taking the pain medication? Consult with your surgeon about alternatives. People react differently to pain medication.

It is important to find a pain medication that works best for YOU!

Remember, pain medication and alcohol don't mix!

Stick to taking your pain medication with food.

Sleep

Sleep can be very challenging after knee replacement for the first few weeks.

Is knee pain waking you up at night?

Sleep is vital to help your recovery; here are my hints:

- Sleep alone. We want to protect the knee as much as possible. Sleeping alone also includes *not* allowing your pets to sleep on the bed with you.

- Do your best to sleep on your back.
- People find sleeping in a recliner very comfortable for the early recovery stage. But if you have a history of back pain, do not sleep in recliners, as it can exacerbate your back pain and will not keep the spine in an ideal position.
- Elevate your knee with a pillow under the *heel* for mild support and elevation.
- If you wake up, gently bend your knee 10–12 times to reduce pain or stiffness.
- Extra pain relief medications at bedtime will help you sleep.
- Take naps whenever you can during the day.

Side sleepers, you may find that a small, squishy pillow between your legs helps you get comfortable.

Safety Tip

When you plan to get out of bed, it is essential to give yourself a moment by counting to 10 as you sit on the side of the bed.

Make sure you feel clear-headed and not dizzy. Give yourself a moment to think about how you will use the walker to stand up and move carefully.

Stairs

If you must climb stairs in your home, the physical therapist at the hospital should have taught you the proper technique and allowed you to practice before going home. When climbing up, you must lead with your nonsurgical leg. But when climbing down stairs, lead with your surgical leg.

If you must use stairs during your first week at home, use a handrail and climb slowly with your nonsurgical knee. If you can avoid them for the first few weeks, it will help reduce your risk of falling.

Absolutely ensure you wear something on your feet so you don't slip on the stairs. And remember—up with the good, down with the bad.

Potty Talk

After surgery, a very common side effect of anesthesia is constipation. Your surgeon may have provided you with instructions to follow to keep this from happening.

If you haven't had a bowel movement on your normal schedule after you get home, you need to take action, as this can become a health risk and reduce the effectiveness of your pain medications.

Drink plenty of fluids. Water is the most desirable choice to aid your digestion. You can also try warmed prunes and warm prune juice.

Increase your fiber intake. Many surgeons will tell you to take fiber supplements when you return home.

Monitor your bowel movements and take stool softeners and/or laxatives to prevent constipation.

Remember, normal bowel movements will aid in a faster, more comfortable recovery, so hydrate, hydrate, hydrate!

Toilet Tips

Many people opt for a toilet riser with handles to make getting up and down easier. Depending on the height of their toilet, this can be an invaluable tool.

After surgery, it's normal to need a device to help you use the toilet. You can find these at medical equipment stores and online. You can find links to some of our specialty item recommendations by scanning the following QR code or going to the "resources" section of thekneezone.com:

thekneezone.com/resources

Another option is a walker with a built-in toilet bucket; use this if you don't want to access a toilet riser.

You can also use your walker as an ad-hoc riser. Simply approach the toilet straight on with your walker. Turn your body around and use the walker handles to help lower yourself. Then, push yourself up again when you want to stand. Finally, maneuver the walker in front of you again to walk.

After surgery, moving on and off the toilet requires strength in your upper body and legs. Be sure to use something to assist you in the bathroom until you feel 100% comfortable with your strength.

Showering Tips

1. If your bandage isn't waterproof, you must protect it from getting wet. Here are a few ways to protect your new knee bandage:
    a. A shower sleeve is handy for people without a waterproof bandage from your surgeon.
    b. Wrap a plastic bag and plastic wrap around your knee.
2. Please use a shower chair and walker to maintain balance and safety.
3. Use a handheld shower attachment if you have one available.
4. Have somebody nearby to help you.
5. If you drop something, leave it and ask someone to help you or bring a grabber in the shower.
6. Take your time, and be mindful of your actions to avoid a possible fall.

You can find links to some of our shower sleeves, shower chairs, and grabber recommendations by scanning the QR code below or going to the "resources" section of thekneezone.com:

thekneezone.com/resources

Do NOT attempt to take a bath, use a spa, or get in a pool!

Trying to take a bath, use a spa, or get in a pool could cause an infection or fall. Do not attempt any of these until your incision has completely healed.

Your surgeon will let you know when it is safe to use the bathtub. **Until then, you should only use the shower.**

Physical Therapy/Exercises

Your surgeon and physical therapist might give you a variety of exercises and devices. What you receive to use might differ from what others receive or what I used during my recovery. Various options should not be a concern to you.

Week 1 is just the beginning of how you commit to yourself and say *yes*, you *will* take care of yourself during your recovery.

I can't emphasize enough that you must work on your recovery *every single day.*

Treat it as your most important job during the next few months.

The good news is that your primary focus for the first two weeks will be straightening your leg. Most surgeons recommend that you do this while icing to minimize swelling.

If you follow the exercise directions, you will recover faster. If you are confused or need help, please don't hesitate to ask for help or clarify what you should be doing. The directions should include how many and how often. Do what you are asked—doing *extra* exercises does not help you heal faster.

Weeks 1 & 2: Your first exercise goal is to straighten that new bionic leg.

You will start hearing the phrase "extension." You will be measured regularly to see how straight you can get your leg. The sooner your leg is straight (full extension), the faster you can bend it further.

You will also hear the phrase "flexion." Knee flexion is the bending of your knee. Many people worry about flexion too early in recovery. When you still have swelling in the knee joint, it limits your range of motion. You will have time to work on your range of motion and reach full flexion.

Key range of motion requirements to help your return to future activities:

70°	Walking without a limp
83°	Climb up the stairs safely
90°	Get in and out of the car
95°	Descend the stairs safely
105°	Rise up from a chair
115°	Peddle a bicycle
125°	Squat
130°	or greater is considered full flexion for most patients

RICE—Rest, Ice, Compression, Elevate

Ice and elevation are key for pain control. Dr. Sinha's physician's assistant, Vangie, explains the importance of pain control this way …

Imagine two fires in your body—pain and healing. If the pain fire is out of control because you're not taking medications as directed or icing/elevating, then all your body's firefighters are trying to put that fire out rather than focusing on healing. But if your pain is controlled, your firefighters can work on putting out the healing fire.

Control the pain so your body can heal.

Setting yourself up for success to reduce swelling and recover optimally will require you to:

- Rest as much as possible; your body needs to recover.
- Ice your new knee. At a minimum, you should ice for 20 minutes every three hours while elevating your leg.
- Keep wearing the compression stockings as directed if they were given to you to wear.
- Elevate your leg. Your toes ideally should be above your nose.
- Leg straightening: do not put a pillow directly under your new knee. Instead, focus on keeping that entire leg as straight as possible.

These five things will be key to your recovery for the next few weeks. You must create a place in your home to sit comfortably and stay on schedule to ice, elevate, and straighten your leg.

The better you stay on schedule, the quicker you will likely recover.

Ice Your New Knee

Most surgeons recommend ice as much as possible during the first two weeks of your recovery. It will reduce the swelling and relieve pain for the next few weeks. As directed by your surgeon, you should keep ice on your new knee.

Every surgeon and region of the world may approach what they recommend differently, as may what your insurance company approves for assistance with icing.

In my case, I got the Game Ready Ice Machine, which had two compression cuffs that, when plugged in and turned on, filled with ice-cold water. The first two weeks, when I was awake, I typically used an ice machine for about 20–30 minutes at a time as needed for swelling and pain. Below is a picture of what that looks like. Achieving this level of elevation is optimal for short periods of time to reduce swelling while icing.

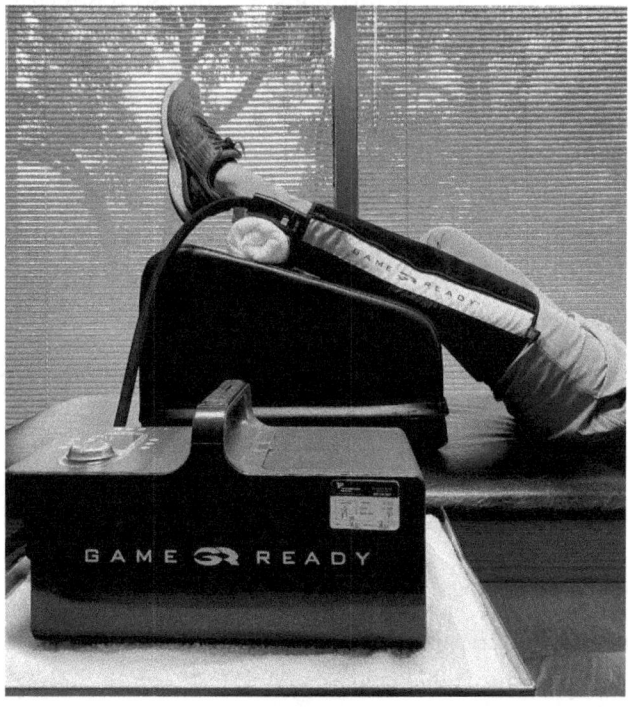

You may have a fancy electric-powered ice machine that will supply cold water via tubes with a velcro wrap around your leg that circulates ice-cold water to use. These machines are very helpful in reducing the time you need to get up or for the people caring for you to help you as frequently.

If your insurance company didn't approve an ice machine and you want one, you can probably rent one, order one from Amazon, possibly find one on Facebook Marketplace, or ask your friends if they have one you can borrow.

You do not need a "fancy" ice machine to have a successful recovery. You must still ice that knee using some method. A plastic bag filled with ice on your knee until it melts and then repeat can work fine—it just takes a little more physical effort from your helpers.

Icing Tips

Do:

- Ensure you have a fabric liner between your ice pack and bare skin with your bandage. I used a pillowcase on mine.
- While you are icing the knee, it is essential to keep it elevated.

Do not:

- Place your ice pack on your bare skin or bandage.

Compression Stockings

When you woke up from surgery, you very likely discovered compression stockings on your feet. These help prevent swelling, improve blood circulation, and reduce the risk of blood clots. Your surgeon will tell you how long you will need to wear them.

Many surgeons recommend wearing them full-time for the first two weeks after surgery. You should leave them on as much as possible, day and night.

Yes, they can be uncomfortable! But getting a blood clot and risking a pulmonary embolism after getting your bionic upgrade isn't worth the risk of not wearing them.

Elevate Your Leg the Right Way

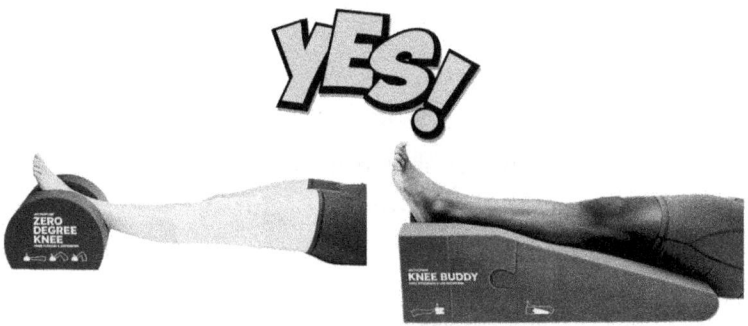

Do:

- Your leg must be elevated from the ankle to your knee with pillows piled up until your toes are above your nose.
- About 20–30 minutes of elevating will help reduce swelling.
- Repeat this 4–6 times a day.
- Make sure your entire leg is elevated, not just your knee.
- Keep your foot flexed (toes pulled toward your face) to help ensure your leg is straight.

Do Not Elevate Your Leg the Wrong Way

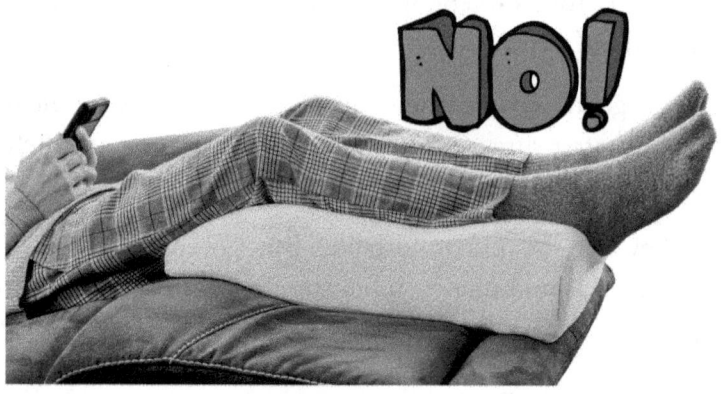

Do Not:

- Keep your leg level or downward—this will increase your swelling and discomfort.
- Bend your knee as shown in the photograph, and have your ankles level or lower than your knee.

Quick Tips to Control Swelling

1. Ice & elevate.
2. Drink water and eat healthy meals.
3. Stretch your knee often.
4. Do your physical therapy exercises as instructed.
5. Don't do too much walking.

What to Do With Your Newfound Time

During the first two weeks of your recovery, you may not feel like doing anything, which is typical for most people.

The first two weeks might be a great time to:

- Listen to a podcast.
- Listen to an audiobook.
- Do Crossword, Sudoku, or other games on your phone.
- Binge-watch a series you have been wanting to see.
- Read this book a few times!

These activities pair well with your main activity: resting, icing, elevating, and straightening.

I started a list on my phone of anything that popped into my mind that I might want to do in future weeks of my recovery, including creating The Knee Zone to help people who are going through knee replacements.

PRO TIP: Turn off the tracking devices.

My friend, you will not reach 10,000 steps for the next two weeks and probably won't close all your exercise goal "rings" for quite some time. If you can't rest at night until you close all three rings on your watch or hit your tracking goals, please take off the device and give yourself the gift of healing.

Don't worry, you will be using them again soon.

Have a Schedule—And Stick With It

During the first two weeks of your recovery period, you will need to stay on your medication schedule.

Having a schedule also means you must do your best to schedule sleep and nap times. Sleep can be very challenging for some people.

If you find staying on a schedule for the first two weeks challenging, setting alarms on your phone or another device to remind you can be helpful.

Write down your schedule and check off your progress. This will help you stay motivated and on track.

An example of a schedule can look like this:

7:00 AM	Wake up, drink a glass of water, and take morning medications that don't require food
7:30 AM	Ice, elevate, and straighten
8:00 AM	Eat breakfast—take medications that require food
8:30 AM	Rest and elevate
9:00 AM	Dress and get ready for the day
9:30 AM	Rest and elevate
10:00 AM	Ice, elevate, and straighten
11:00 AM	Take a break and do something on your "new-found time list"
12:00 PM	Lunch and take medications
1:00 PM	Ice, elevate, and straighten
2:00 PM	Rest and elevate

3:00 PM	Take a break and do something on your "new-found time list"
4:00 PM	Afternoon medications with snack
5:00 PM	Physical therapy exercises
6:00 PM	Ice, elevate, & straightening
7:00 PM	Dinner and take medications
8:00 PM	Rest and elevate
9:00 PM	Take a break and do something on your "new-found time list"
10:00 PM	Ice, elevate, and straighten
10:30 PM	Get ready for bed—last medication review of the day
11:00 PM	Go to sleep
Overnight	Ice as needed

Wow, you are going to be busy! Your schedule can change radically based on many factors, which is okay. However, you need a written daily schedule to track and check your progress.

Please make a daily schedule for yourself that contains these key things:

1. Take your medications on schedule.
2. Fuel your body—your body needs good nutrition to recover. Many people become malnourished after knee replacement surgery, but not you! You'll want to increase your healthy protein intake after surgery to maintain muscle mass, support bone health, enhance immune function, and promote healing.

3. Ice, elevate, and straighten your leg with your toes above your nose.
4. Take rest breaks—if you take a nap, that is a bonus. Please note that naps can interfere with nighttime sleep, so you should be mindful of how long you nap during the day.
5. Do some sort of physical therapy daily. Depending on what your surgeon and/or physical therapist suggest, you may do things more than once a day.

Low Furniture

Take a look at the height of the furniture in your home. If your favorite chair requires a deep knee bend to sit down, you will find it extremely difficult to stand up later.

Find a chair to sit on, preferably with arms on it, to help you lower down and push yourself up. If your sofa is too low to sit on, try stacking cushions or piling some pillows to raise the seat height.

To elevate your leg, find something you can have someone move in front of the chair and pile on pillows to get the elevation you need. Remember, your toes need to be higher than your nose.

If your furniture has deep cushions, push yourself to the edge with your legs comfortably bent and touching the floor, then stand with help from your walker or chair arms.

Diana's Story: An Encounter with a Low Sofa

During the first two weeks of my recovery, we stayed at a beautiful rental property in Arizona. When we returned from the hospital, I chose a bedroom close to the living room with a bathroom attached that would be easy for me to access without many steps.

When I ventured out to the living room to sit on the beautiful sofa, I quickly realized that getting up would require some major effort—in my case, my husband hoisted me up. We quickly decided I wouldn't sit on that sofa again during our stay.

My new seat was a heavy wrought-iron patio chair with armrests, a big cushion, and an ottoman on which we could pile pillows high enough to ensure my legs were properly elevated.

Hopefully, you won't require assistance or hoisting to get up like I did.

*Be sure to look at the height of things **before** you sit on them. For the first two weeks, the higher the chair, the better.*

Tip: You can always pile pillows or double seat cushions to increase your height, making it easier to stand as you recover.

Skin Irritation and Reactions

Your body has had a traumatic experience. It may react in many ways. The medications you take, which are perfectly on schedule, may also cause unwelcome reactions.

If you experience unwanted reactions to medication, such as diarrhea, nausea, vomiting, severe stomach pain, or severe headaches, you should contact your surgeon's office immediately and discuss alternative medications.

I experienced very uncomfortable skin irritation. I suggest you moisturize your skin well—something else that is great to do with your spare time. If you need help getting it on your back, ask for help.

Your scar will be itchy, which means it is healing. Do NOT apply anything to the incision until every scab has fallen off naturally.

Hot knee? Is your skin feeling hot to the touch on your new knee area? This "hot knee" was a discovery I had at about 3 a.m. on my second night home from the hospital.

The trauma of surgery causes increased blood flow to the knee, resulting in a "hot" sensation. This is normal. It can last several months—even up to a year. Keep on icing!

While a certain amount of warmth on the knee is to be expected, you should be concerned when:

- You see a rash next to your adhesive bandage.
- You see non-bloody liquid seeping from the edges of the bandage.
- You have a temperature greater than 101.5^0 F (38.6^0 C) associated with increased pain and heat on the knee.

These could be signs of a possible infection. If you should experience these symptoms, immediately phone your surgeon's office. They will likely schedule a telehealth appointment with you or have you come in right away to take a look.

Leaving the House

As I've repeatedly mentioned, the first two weeks of recovery are best spent at home resting, icing, elevating, and doing physical therapy exercises.

If you need to leave the house for physical therapy or to see your surgeon, please give yourself ample time to get ready. Consider what clothing and shoes will be comfortable and functional. Make sure you have your walker and give yourself plenty of time to get into the car.

As a refresher, quickly review my guide to getting in and out of the car:

1. Be sure the vehicle's height is manageable—getting into a lifted truck or a low sports car will be really difficult.
2. Position the front passenger seat as far back as possible.
3. Put the window down and open the door as wide as you can.
4. Approach the passenger seat with your back facing the seat by carefully using your walker.
5. Back up gently until you feel the car right behind you.
6. Let the driver take your walker away while you hold the car door.
7. Keep your bionic leg a step forward and hold on to the windowsill and car frame for support.

8. Slowly bend your head and chest forward, sticking your bottom out until it makes contact with the seat. Sigh with relief.
9. Watch your head and slide onto the seat securely.
10. Slowly turn toward the front of the car and lift one leg in after the other. At first, you may need to help lift your bionic leg into the car.
11. Sit forward, exhale, and remind yourself this will get easier each time. Then, close the door, and off you go.

Remember, leather can stick to your skin in warm weather. If you stick to the seat and it is hard to turn, you can put a plastic garbage bag or towel on the seat to help you turn more easily.

Also, if you are tall and stretching your bionic leg is difficult, you can sit sideways on a bench seat in the back until you improve your range of motion.

Mental Health Check-In

Give yourself grace these first two weeks of recovery. Your body has undergone a major surgery.

You might feel exhausted, sad, angry, or lonely.

Please ensure you are reaching out to positive people in your life for a pep talk. Many people may not be reaching out to you because they don't want to disturb your rest. Now is the time for you to call them for support.

For a quick reference guide for Weeks 1 & 2 of your recovery, check out:

thekneezone.com/recoveryguides

Dr. Sinha's Recommendations for Weeks 1 & 2

Once you're home, there are several key aspects to recovery. As I mentioned before, controlling pain in the first few days is critical because the more effectively you use the pain medication early on, the less overall pain medication you're going to need throughout your recovery.

Said another way, the better you control your pain early on, the less pain medication you will need later on.

Said yet another way, if you try to tough it out early on, you will not do well later on. There is no reward for suffering. People are often fearful of getting addicted to narcotics. You will not get addicted in the first two weeks. It doesn't work that way, and if you're in my practice, I won't let you get addicted at all because if you're exhibiting addictive behavior, there are ways that I can put a stop to that.

The most important thing I want you to do in the first week or so is to get the knee fully extended (straight). When you have arthritis, the knee feels better when it's slightly bent, so during that whole period that the knee is degenerating, you subconsciously keep it bent a little bit and then a little bit more over time. Some people get to a point where they can't even fully straighten the knee out because all the tissues around it become contracted (shortened).

At the time of surgery, we straighten your leg all the way out. We release the necessary tissues and reach the point where the knee is entirely straight because that's a critical component of the operation and your recovery.

But after surgery, it may still feel better when bent, so when you get home, you will be tempted to put a pillow under it and bend it. ***That is a big no-no.*** Put the pillow under your heel and keep the knee straightened out because the quicker you get it (or keep it) straight, the quicker it flexes and the less pain you'll have.

The other common misconception is that pain occurs primarily inside the knee. Still, it's interesting that most of the pain you experience is caused by swelling in the leg rather than from the incision or even the work we do inside the bone. It's the swelling that causes the pain.

Not having great muscle tissue in your calves before surgery makes you prone to swelling in your feet and ankles. The swelling below your knee will actually create more discomfort than the pain from your knee. That's why it's so important to not only ice the surgical site but also elevate the entire leg. In fact, that's your primary job in the first week: ice, elevate, and keep the swelling down to help limit the pain.

And, of course, get your knee fully straight.

You'll also be given a series of exercises to do, and you'll have instructions on how often to do them. Please, please, please follow the instructions.

You get no value from doing more exercise early on because biology, being biology, will move on its own timeline. You can't do anything to speed that timeline up. All you can do is slow the timeline down by doing stupid things, and Daddy used to say, "Stupid should hurt."

What about the bandage? Most surgeons now use waterproof bandages because one of the big things patients talked to us about was the ability to shower after surgery. They felt icky and wanted to shower, so we developed waterproof bandages.

You can't submerge the leg in a bath, a hot tub, or a pool early on, but you can certainly shower. That bandage should not be removed because the incision is the cleanest and most sterile when the operation is finished. Plus, the bandage may have an antimicrobial layer designed to prevent infection.

Most of these bandages are designed to stay on between 7 and 14 days, depending on the surgeon's protocol. You can shower over them, but leave them be. You can ice over the bandages as they are designed to allow cooling to pass through. A lot of them will actually wick blood away from the incision.

We don't want the incision to be wet, so if you see blood on the bandage, that's not anything to panic about. That's actually a good thing, as these bandages are designed to pull the blood away from the skin.

You should start to be concerned if blood begins to leak *outside* the edge of the bandage. Then, you need to be evaluated. But as long as the blood stays contained within the absorbent part of the bandage, all is good.

Sleep after surgery, or lack thereof. It's a relatively new phenomenon. I would say 30 years ago, when I started practice, we only had one way to control pain after surgery, and that was with opioids. And guess what? Opioids knock you out.

In the first 10 years of my practice, I never heard a person complain about not being able to sleep after surgery because they were taking so many opioids. They slept most of the day and night, as it turned out.

But as we started moving toward fewer opioids, more regional pain management, and other non-narcotic medications, sleep became more of an issue. And what I hear patients tell me is that they can't find a position to get comfortable. It's not like they hurt during the day; they just ache at night. A common question is, "Why don't I hurt when I'm moving? But when I stop moving, suddenly I hurt."

The answer has to do with muscles. You're using your muscles all day long. Remember, these muscles were weak before the surgery due to longstanding arthritis, atrophy, and all that stuff I've already discussed.

After being used all day, they ache at the end of the day. And that's what keeps you awake. The best thing from a muscle standpoint is anti-inflammatory medications (such as ibuprofen, naproxen, celecoxib, meloxicam, or, in some cases, low-dose steroids). If you can take anti-inflammatories, that would be very helpful.

In terms of sleeping pills, it's okay to use them. You can also use melatonin for a few weeks after surgery. If you use something like zolpidem (trade name Ambien), you don't want to use it for more than two or three weeks after surgery.

If you rely on opioids to help you sleep, they will help you fall asleep. However, your sleep quality is not as restful as if you fell asleep with a sleeping aid like melatonin, zolpidem, or one of those related medications.

You will read elsewhere in this book about how important it is to get sleep and some tips and tricks you can try. Pharmacologically, starting to load up on anti-inflammatories around dinnertime should help you sleep.

A glass of wine is OK. **One** glass, not a bottle. And when I say one, I mean a standard glass, not the kind of glass you can pour a whole bottle into.

Key Takeaways for Weeks 1 & 2 of Recovery

1. Positive Mindset
   - It is critical that you remember that you are starting a new chapter of your life after your surgery.
   - From the moment your eyes pop open in the morning, you should remind yourself that you are another day into your recovery and grateful to live in this modern world where we can get new body parts.
   - You are on your way to becoming stronger, faster, and better, like the Bionic Man or Woman of the modern day.
2. Rest, ice, compression, elevate, and focus on straightening your leg.
3. For a quick reference guide for your first two weeks of recovery that you can print out and keep handy, go to:

thekneezone.com/recoveryguides

RECOVERY GUIDE
WHAT TO EXPECT
WEEKS 2–4

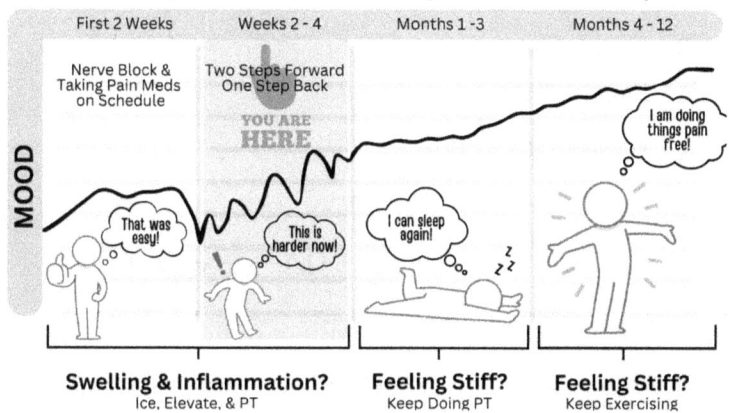

For most people, Weeks 2–4 can be the most challenging part of their recovery. A game plan for coping and knowing what to expect will make the next two weeks manageable.

I have coached people through these next two weeks, and I promise you are making progress even if your perceived lack of progress suggests otherwise. This is the two steps forward, one step back zone for many during recovery.

Here are the key things for Weeks 2–4 and how to help manage them:

1. Sleep
2. Mental Health Check-In
3. Surgeon Visit
4. Pain & Swelling
5. Scar Care
6. Sensitivity & Itching = Healing
7. Numbness on Your Knee
8. Physical Therapy
9. Going Out
10. Dental Work
11. Returning to Work

Sleep

How has sleeping been for you the last two weeks?

Great, good, OK, or "what is sleep"?

Some fall into the "what is sleep" category—I'm your people!

I'm so happy for you if you are in the "great or good" category. You are getting the energy you need to heal.

If you are in the "OK" or "what is sleep" category, it is time to figure out what prevents you from sleeping.

Here are some tips:

- You will likely have better luck sleeping alone in bed a little longer.
- Having a dark, cool, quiet room will help.
- Consider trying Melatonin or another sleep aid.

- Don't allow your pets to sleep on the bed with you. Have them visit you during the daytime.

Is pain waking you up at night?

- Make sure you ice before trying to fall asleep.
- Time pain medication as late as possible.
- Experiment with physical therapy exercises before bed to ensure you loosen up your new knee.
- Elevate your leg with a pillow for MILD support and elevation.
- If you wake up, gently bend your knee 10-12 times to reduce pain or stiffness.
- Try a heating pad on your quad muscles for 15 minutes before bed.

Sleeping Positions:

Do your best to sleep on your back.

For the first few weeks, sleeping in a recliner can be very comfortable. However, if you have a history of back pain, do not sleep in recliners, as they can exacerbate the pain and do not keep the spine in an ideal position.

Side sleepers: As you enter this recovery phase, you will likely find sleeping longer easier. Experiment with a squishy, small pillow between your legs to help you get comfortable.

Tip: If you have an airplane neck pillow, try placing it between your legs to relieve pressure.

Please remember: When you get out of bed, it is important to give yourself a moment to sit on the side of the bed and count down from 10 to 1 before you stand up.

Make sure you feel clear-headed and not dizzy. Give yourself a moment to think about how you will stand up and move carefully.

Mental Health Check-In

It is very common for the next two weeks to feel emotionally difficult.

You might feel frustrated, regretful, sad, angry, and shed a tear due to fatigue, cabin fever, pain, and frustration over your perceived lack of progress.

Deep breaths, friend!

Tips:

- Get some fresh air! Sit outside and take in a different view!
- Talk—yes, talk, not text—with your friends and family.
- Please ensure you are reaching out to positive people in your life for a pep talk. Many people may not be reaching out to you because they don't want to disturb your rest. Now is the time for you to call them for support.
- Start a journal of your daily wins! What is something you did today you couldn't do two weeks ago?

You are only a few weeks into a complete recovery that can take up to a year. Don't let that scare you; it is information that will provide you with perspective.

You wouldn't expect a newborn to be able to climb a flight of stairs, shower, and sleep easily. Let that baby knee have time to mature.

Surgeon Visit

You will likely visit your surgeon or a staff member during this time.

The night before your surgeon's visit, make a list of all your questions. Be sure to bring your list with you and write down the answers. It is easy to forget what you hear; writing it down will help you remember.

Questions You Might Have for Your Surgeon

1. What can I do differently to manage my pain?
2. I'm having issues with sleeping. Is there something that will help me sleep better?
3. Is it normal to experience severe swelling or skin irritation? (Spoiler Alert: it's not normal, so you need to let them know ASAP.)
4. How should I care for my wound now that I can see it?

You can expect a few things during this visit. For example:

- You may get approval to stop wearing the compression stockings.
- You might get sutures, skin staples, zipline, or tape strips removed. You may have sterile tape strips placed over the wound after suture removal. It is important to follow the directions your surgeon provides you to care for your wound.
- You could get X-rays.
- Your surgeon may allow you to see your X-rays and even possibly take a picture of them to show friends and family your bionic upgrade.

- You will walk around and show off how great your recovery is going.
- You should have your flexion and extension measured. Jot down those numbers so you can track your progress.

Most people experience pain relief after their bandage and sutures are removed because they can move their knee more easily.

Pain & Swelling

You are entering the recovery phase, allowing you to walk around more. You may find yourself walking around the house without a walker and moving to a cane. Hurray! Another step in your recovery! But this newfound freedom from assistive devices often comes with swelling, soreness, and maybe pain.

Key things:
- Swelling will increase with activity.
- Do the necessary tasks in the morning when you have the least swelling.
- Ice, elevate, and straighten immediately after you complete tasks.
- You may feel terrific and "overdo" it. If you do too much, it will result in more pain and swelling. You must experiment to find your sweet spot for activity time on your feet.
- You will be sore daily—this will decrease over time.
- Your new knee may feel hot to the touch—this is normal.
- If you feel ready to use the cane, ask your physical therapist for help to learn the proper techniques and start practicing with it.

Scar Care

Once the bandages and sutures are removed from your new knee, you might immediately wonder what you can put on the scars to make them look better.

The answer is NOTHING YET!

You do not want to get an infection. You have come too far in your recovery to risk going back to surgery with an infection, which could potentially result in that new knee being replaced all over again.

Do not risk getting an infection.

Tips:

- Don't put anything on the wound unless your surgeon prescribes or approves it.
- Dr. Google is not your surgeon.
- Nurse Chat GPT is not qualified either.
- Avoid touching the scabs.
- Do not let a pet lick your wounds.
- Do not enter a swimming pool, spa, or bathtub.

I promise that we will focus on scar care once the scar is fully closed and the scabs are gone.

Sensitivity & Itching = Healing

Once the bandage and stitches are removed, you will likely notice that anything touching your knee is uncomfortable. Also, you may feel a pins and needles sensation as the skin nerves heal and come back to life.

- Icing more throughout the day will help. Try a bag of frozen peas with a paper towel barrier or a postoperative gel pack. The therapy wrap from CoolJaw.com is hands-free, comfortable, and doesn't leak.
- Start putting fabric on the knee, and start with loose, soft fabrics. We will work our way up to denim.
- Massage your knee to help desensitize it and break up scar tissue.

Numbness on Your Knee

When you have your knee replaced, your skin is cut. Skin nerves are also cut during your surgery. This leads to initial numbness along the incision. You will likely notice the numbness, especially once the nerves begin to heal and come back to life. This is the pins and needles sensation phase.

A small number of people will have a small patch of permanent numbness on the outer side of the knee. Over time, the size of that patch shrinks to the size of a quarter. According to Dr. Sinha, the area of numbness will not prevent you from a full recovery.

Physical Therapy

Your mobility begins to improve considerably during this recovery phase. Yes, you will still be doing your exercises daily.

You will begin walking further each day and SLOWLY increase the distance day by day.

As you improve, your physical therapist will continue introducing you to new exercises, some of which will challenge you. This is not the point to stop pushing yourself. Yes, it is hard work. Don't give up. Keep trying a little more each day.

And don't despair! You are teaching that new knee these moves for the first time.

If you can access a foot peddler, recumbent bike, or another PT-type bike, you can improve your range of motion using these devices. Be careful as you use them, and don't overdo it. You are not training for the Tour de France. Start by using it for a few minutes and *slowly* increase the time you use it.

Perform your physical therapy exercises daily, as provided by your physical therapist. If you have a "setback" day, it is OK— but make sure you try your best again the next day. You don't want to regress in your range of motion or straightening.

If you can work with multiple therapists, having others observe and teach you different exercises can be helpful.

Going Out

This is the point at which you might feel ready to venture out into the world again.

Tips:

- Give yourself plenty of time to get ready to venture out.
- If you plan to be in a car for over two hours, you must stop and take a break.
- Once you arrive and get out of the car, be sure to stretch and walk for five minutes. You will likely feel stiff from any time in the car.
- If you notice swelling in your new knee, keep a plastic bag with you if you need to ice it. Having a bag handy to fill with ice from a small ice chest is helpful.

- Bring your walker if you encounter a low toilet and need help getting up or down. It can also help you with chairs.
- Know the parking situation—how far will you need to walk, and will you need to deal with steps?
- Know the seating situation—Can you stretch out your leg? What is the height of the chairs?

> ### Diana's Story: Walkers Aren't Just for Walking
>
> *A few weeks after my surgery, I attended a Thanksgiving dinner with family. During the festivities, I made it a point to sit, ice, and elevate.*
>
> *I also thought ahead and brought my walker with me—not because I needed it to help me keep my balance while walking, but to help me with sitting and standing. I am beyond grateful I had it to lean on.*
>
> *The walker helped me lower myself and get up from another beautiful low sofa. And do you know what made it an absolute lifesaver? Bringing it with me to the guest toilet. There's nothing quite like firsthand experience!*
>
> *Remember, I had both my knees replaced simultaneously, so your outings might be easier than mine were early in recovery.*

Dental Work

After knee replacement surgery, most surgeons and dentists recommend preventative antibiotics for both routine and emergency dental work. This is usually one dose taken one hour before your appointment.

The antibiotic you're prescribed by your surgeon will vary based on your medical history, including allergies. A single dose could be from one up to four pills that you take all at once. Otherwise, you could risk an infection of your new knee. Please tell your dentist's office you had a knee replacement when making the appointment.

If you have an urgent dental need before the six-week mark of your recovery, it is even more critical to remember you need an antibiotic in advance. Reminder: It is crucial to take the pills one hour ***before*** your appointment.

Returning to Work

Depending on your work type, you can return to work sooner if you work remotely from home on a laptop vs. standing on your feet most of the day. I thought I was "ready" to return to work early, and I was wrong!

Many people take at least six weeks off before going back to work. The type of work you do can drastically change your return-to-work status. Someone like me, who works from home full time and can move around easily to elevate and ice, can return to work earlier than somebody with a physically demanding or tasking job (like a roofer or a retail clerk).

Speak to your surgeon about the type of work you do and what amount of time off seems reasonable for your recovery.

You must also be aware of your emotional state and honest with your co-workers. You just had a bionic upgrade, and it is a long and significant recovery.

If you don't sleep well every night, you cannot regain 100% of your energy. I was shocked by my fatigue after working just a few hours. I found it nearly impossible to get comfortable.

If you return to work at this point, I urge you to make sure your co-workers understand you are returning "early" and that you still need to take daily physical therapy breaks. Ideally, you should work part-time if possible and build up to full-time hours as you feel able.

Keep your mind on what you want to happen, not what you don't want to have happen.

Diana's Story: A Cautionary Tale

A few weeks after my bilateral knee replacements, I was home "unsupervised" and feeling ready to do more around the house. The truth is, I was going a little stir-crazy and thought I could do something more valuable than journaling, reading, and using my physical therapy bike.

I thought I could easily change the sheets on our king-size bed, which was wrong. I didn't consider the amount of bending, turning, and stretching involved with that task ahead of time. Eventually, my right foot started to pivot and twist, and I didn't have the quad strength to stop sliding. Luckily, I flopped face down on the bed, not the floor.

I was angry and in pain—I may have shed a tear or two. After that, it took me three days of resting, icing, and elevating to recover. I'm sharing this humiliation with you so you understand why I became passionate about helping others avoid having a setback. That is how I began creating The Knee Zone.

For a quick reference guide of Weeks 2–4 that you can print out and keep handy, go to:

thekneezone.com/recoveryguides

> **Dr. Sinha's Point of View: What You Should Expect During That First Visit**
>
> Every surgeon has a protocol for following up with patients. For example, my protocol is to have the patients come in at one week, two weeks, and six weeks.
>
> The one-week visit is basically to ensure that the bandage looks OK, that you're doing what you're supposed to be doing, that your swelling is controlled, that you're working on getting the knee straight, and that you're not worrying too much about the bending.
>
> On the second visit, we remove the bandage. Currently, I use skin glue with zip ties that pull the skin together so there are no sutures or staples. The advantage is that when you take the bandage off, those zip ties just peel right off the skin, which is pretty pain-free. But the other advantage is that because there's nothing in the skin, the incisions look better in the long term.

I get an X-ray at the two-week point to ensure that nothing undesirable is happening to the implant. At that point, I'll make decisions about changing you from home physical therapy to outpatient physical therapy, cutting back on your therapy, or ramping up on your therapy, all depending upon how your knee looks, moves, and feels.

If you followed my instructions those first two weeks, you'll feel pretty good at the two-week mark. You'll be off your narcotics. You'll be pretty much getting by with acetaminophen and an anti-inflammatory medication. I can always tell when people haven't followed the instructions because they need more narcotics.

The six-week visit: I want to ensure you've hit certain milestones. Certainly, I want that knee fully straight, and I want you to bend it to at least 90 degrees.

If you're only at 90 degrees, it's no reason to panic. If you're way beyond 90 degrees, that's also no reason to panic. Remember, there are no awards here. This is not a competition.

Everybody progresses at their own pace, and my staff and I will adjust your post-op protocols to ensure that you're moving in the proper direction and accomplishing the goals you want and need to achieve.

Once you've hit the six-week point and you're looking good, and if everything's going smoothly, I probably won't see you again for another two months. During that two-month interval, you'll hopefully complete physical therapy and increase your activities. When I see you at the three-and-a-half-month point, I'll remove all restrictions if everything has gone well and you've met the appropriate goals.

Key Takeaways for Weeks 2–4 of Recovery

1. **Progress isn't linear—stay patient**
   - Recovery feels like two steps forward, one step back. Expect ups and downs.
2. **Manage sleep, pain, and swelling**
   - Optimize sleep environment, time meds, and ice before bed.
   - Balance activity with rest—overdoing it leads to setbacks.
3. **Mental and emotional well-being matter**
   - Frustration and fatigue are normal—get fresh air, talk to supportive people, and track small wins.
4. **Follow surgeon and PT guidance**
   - Ask about pain management, track flexion/extension, and be cautious with scar care.
   - Continue PT exercises daily—gradually increase mobility by walking a little further each day.
5. **Plan outings and work carefully**
   - Consider seating, walking distance, and swelling when going out.
   - Ease back into work if possible—fatigue is real, and recovery takes time.

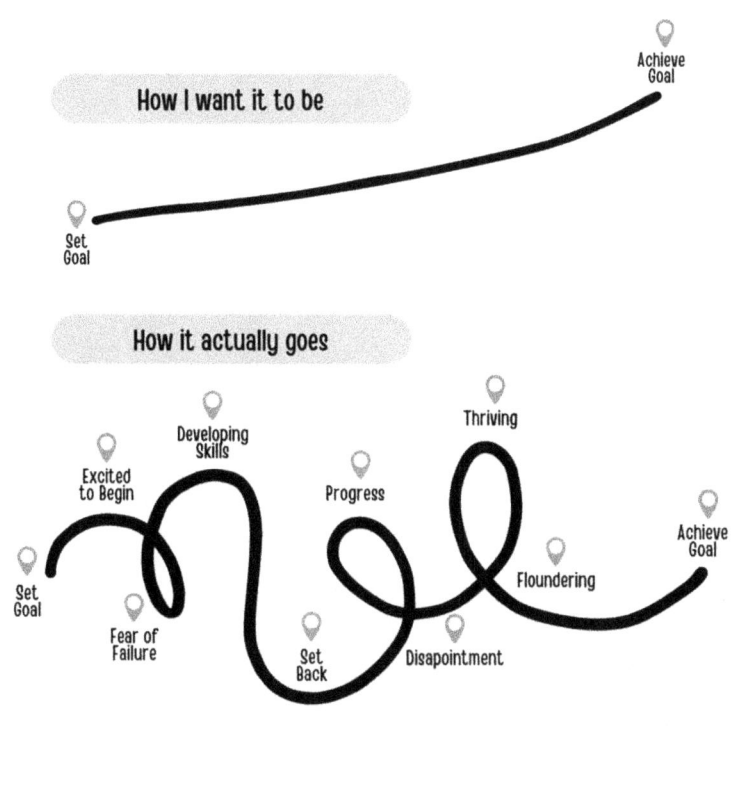

MONTHS 1 & 2
GETTING OUT INTO THE WORLD

Celebrate Your Progress!

Congratulations, you have made it past your first month kneeversary. Remember, this recovery can take up to a year. Staying consistent with your recovery efforts is critical to help you recover faster and return to thriving.

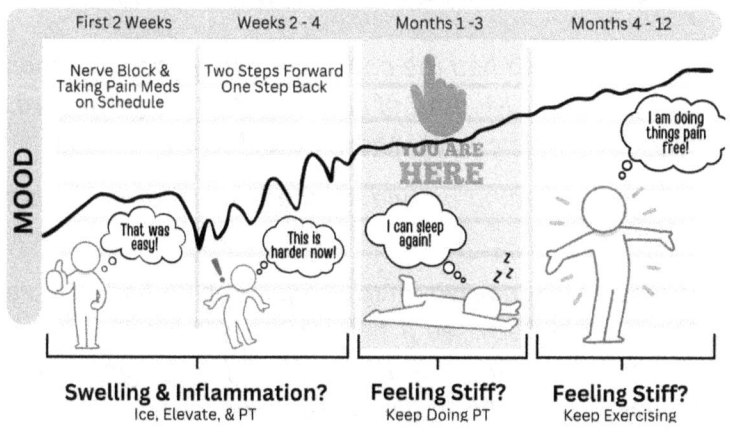

Progress is not linear; for some, it may require two steps backward before you can take a big leap forward. I certainly experienced this during my recovery in the first year.

As you enter your second month of recovery, you must celebrate your WINS!

1. Look at your improvement in straightening and range of motion in the last four weeks! By now, you are likely at or surpassing 90-degree bending.
2. If you have strengthened your quad muscles enough, you can move around the house without canes or walkers.

Braving the Outside World

Around the second month of recovery, the people I coach start asking me questions about how to go on trips safely. In this section, I'll share some tips for safely resuming activities.

> ### Diana's Story of a Client Who Was "Bummed Out"
>
> *A client I coached had the opportunity to go on a pontoon boat ride around Month 2 of recovery. We thought she was ready. So away she went. Ahoy, Matey!*
>
> *Challenge 1. Getting on and off the boat on a rocky dock was scary.*
>
> *Challenge 2. The ride was much longer than we had planned when we had discussed it beforehand. During the ride, it was potty time—and the potty was a five-gallon bucket. She found it very challenging to squat on that.*
>
> *Luckily, a friend was willing to help hold up a towel for privacy and an arm for balancing.*

Weather Conditions Changing?

Your knee will tell you if the weather is changing by suddenly feeling stiff and causing joint pain during the early phases of your recovery.

When the weather changes, barometric pressure can drop, causing the tissues around your joints to expand. This tissue expansion puts further pressure on the joint that is recovering.

The stiffness reaction diminishes over time as you recover—but hey, you can add "weather forecaster" to your list of special skills to impress your friends and family after your bionic upgrade.

Driving Trips (Longer Than 3 Hours)

1. Always bring an empty gallon Ziplock bag if you need ice on the go. Consider taking along a small ice chest.
2. Be sure to stop on your drive to get out of the car, walk around, and stretch.
3. You should stop every 2–3 hours; otherwise, you will become very stiff when you attempt to leave the car and walk again.
4. Sitting in the back seat sideways might be more comfortable for part of your drive, allowing you to stretch out.
5. Move your leg as much as possible with mini foot pumps and leg lifts to prevent stiffness.
6. If you start noticing swelling or discomfort, grab the plastic bag you are traveling with, fill it with ice, and place it on your knee.

Visiting New Places

Once you are outside your house visiting new places, you will encounter new things that you will want to navigate carefully.

1. Always bring an empty gallon Ziplock bag if you need ice on the go.
2. Check the height of things BEFORE you sit down to ensure you can easily get on and off a chair, bed, or sofa. If they are too low, you can pile pillows to reach a safer height.
3. Be careful of cords, rugs, and bumpy surfaces—slow and steady wins recovery.
4. Bring your walker to be 100% safe. You want to be able to get up and down in any bathroom situation easily, and it is good protection if you are in a crowded place.
5. Pack a heating pad for the back of your knee, side of your leg from hip to knee (your IT band), and quad or calf muscles to help combat stiffness from driving or extra walking.
6. Ice, of course, is still the best friend of that new bionic upgrade.
7. How far will you be walking that day? Are you ready?
8. What is the terrain? Gravel, steps, slopes, and weather (please, no dancing in the rain yet).
9. Take anti-inflammatory pain relief medicine on schedule that day and bring extras with you—I learned this lesson the hard way. Please learn from my experience.

Stairs

It is time to start making friends with stairs again. I despised stairs before my surgery.

Now I know I can use them pain-free *and* worry-free!

1. Stairs—The easy way to go up or down stairs is to use your nonsurgical leg as the lead—to get in some new PT moves, you do the opposite. Here is a link to a video I made that hopefully helps you:

   thekneezone.com/education

2. Stretching on stairs: You will have a GREAT opportunity to do some gentle lunges on the stairs, which can significantly improve your range of motion.

3. Continue working your steps by leading with the surgical leg—probably something you haven't done in years. It will build your confidence.

Scar Care

- You are ready for scar care if all the scabs are gone from your incision. This can occur anywhere from 4–6 weeks after your surgery.
- Things you can try are plentiful on the market:
  o Mederma (or store brand)
  o Vitamin E oil
  o Scar strips
- Massaging around the scar will also reduce itching.
- Avoid sun exposure during this phase of recovery to prevent your scars from becoming darker and slower to heal. After one year, your scar can handle more sun exposure.

Pedicures

I wanted a pedicure about six weeks after my surgery and discovered some precautions needed to be taken.

My surgeon advised me to wait six weeks post-op before getting one, so I waited as instructed.

I was told if the pedicure draws blood, to take a dose of antibiotics as soon as possible. You should have the antibiotics with you.

Again, I'm not willing to risk getting an infection, and I hope you won't risk it either. A cut on your foot could risk an infection of your new knee.

Day-to-Day Life—Month 2 Kneeversary

Please remember, everybody is on a different timeline!

You might be further down your path of recovery or still need time to prepare to take on more. For most people, total recovery is a 12-month plan.

Fear not if you aren't ready yet for some of these next steps. This will still provide the insights you need to recover quicker and thrive when you feel ready!

- Get access to a recumbent or stationary bike, and once on it, try pedaling backward a little to see how that feels. It will help you build a greater range of motion and wake up the quad muscles.
- Quad strengthening—this is super important. Try everything and anything to increase your quad strength. The stronger your quad muscles, the faster you will regain range of motion and extension.

- Try to walk more often on uneven surfaces—take it slowly, carefully, and mindfully.
- Step up and down on a step facing forward and sideways.
- Think of engaging your quad muscle every step of heel, toe, heel, toe, heel, toe as you walk.

Sleepy quad in the morning? Here are a few things to try:
- Five minutes of quad strengthening—squats, lunges, stair climbing.
- Make sure you are conscious of "firing" that quad muscle. Achieve firing your quad by actively contracting and by consciously focusing on squeezing the muscles to feel them.
- For an example of how to strengthen your quads using an exercise band, check out the "Quad Strengthening Sitting in a Chair" video at:

    thekneezone.com/education

- Stationary biking, of course! Increase the resistance every minute after a one-minute warm-up. Can you go for 10 minutes?
- Using a TENS unit on your quad muscles can also help. Electric stimulation from a TENS unit is helpful for quad muscle activation, muscle relaxation, and pain management. You can ask your physical therapist about this or purchase one online for home use.

• Challenge yourself by asking your physical therapist for more tips.

- You could go to a store and push a shopping cart to experience the outside world.
- If you feel comfortable, get outside and walk a little daily. Gradually add more steps, but don't expect to walk a few miles on your first few days.
- Make it a point to record things that are becoming easier for you: putting on shoes might be the win of the day, or standing in the kitchen or laundry room completing short tasks.

Pain or Feeling Stiff?

- Mind over matter—You may feel stiff and sore, but you are likely not in pain at this point in your recovery. If you catch yourself saying "pain," check in and ask yourself if it genuinely is pain or if you are "stiff." This mindset transition is vital to helping you heal.
- Icing—Once you start icing your incision, I suggest covering it with a dish towel or pillowcase so you don't irritate that area.
- Try a heating pad behind your knee where that tendon is stiff—you can also massage it a bit.
- Keep massaging your knee to break up the scar tissue and desensitize the area further. Massage your knee area, hamstrings, and quads. This is when a handheld massager can be very helpful when starting daily use.
- It's time to be brave, wear different clothing, and continue desensitizing that knee to "touch."
    - Jeans are the final frontier—it could take a few more months until they feel comfortable against your healing incision.

Zinger Sensations or Heat Near the Incision?

Zinger sensations might begin to occur around this time. They are quick bursts of sharp pricks, like an electric shock around the knee. I thought of these as the nerves colliding with one another, working to get reacquainted.

- This is normal and can last for months.
- The zinger sensations will come and go.
- Inflammation can cause pain, zingers, burning, and swelling, which are common after knee replacement.
- Micro-tears of scar tissue can occur after surgery if you or a physical therapist is giving you too many exercises too soon in your recovery.
- Remember, all those skin nerves in your knee were cut during the surgery, and they are eagerly working to repair themselves.

No! My Knee Does Hurt—It Isn't Just Stiff

You may still have days when you accidentally do too much and feel pain again. During this phase of recovery, you might engage in more and more activity. This may lead to experiencing pain when you accidentally overdo it.

For the days it isn't just stiff, and you label it "pain," try some of the following pain-relief methods:

- Elevate—toes over your nose—roll up a towel and place it under that ankle for extra straightening, and flex your foot as much as you can tolerate. Start a few minutes at a time; it will not feel great.

- Keep icing and give it a rest. You did some major new activities, and even sitting in the car for over an hour is a new experience that can cause stiffness that will hit the tendon, hamstring, and the new bionic upgrade.
- Heating pad—experiment using this on your quad, calf, and behind your knee to reduce the pain.
- Apply Bio-Freeze or Voltaren arthritis cream to your knee's sore tendon and side. **Do not place the cream directly on your incision.**
- Massage, massage, massage—it will break up the tension. A few minutes at a time should give you relief. Consider a massage from a professional, you deserve it!

Projects Around the House

You will likely feel it is time to tackle some projects around the house.

Do's

- Start on projects by setting a timer if you stand up and move around.
- I started with 15 minutes of movement and five minutes of sitting, icing, and straightening. I increased by five minutes daily until I was up to 45 minutes moving and 15 minutes resting.
- At this point, it's great to start tackling your long-awaited list of organizing things around the house, such as kitchen cabinets, the laundry room, the pantry, closets, office files, and any other small tasks you may have in mind that you can do safely.

Don'ts

- Don't forget to set a timer and SLOWLY increase the time you are on your feet.
- Don't pick activities that require you to climb a ladder.
- Don't pick activities that require you to squat down for an extended time.
- Don't pick activities that require you to get down on the ground.

Action Items to Improve Sleep

- If you find sleeping challenging now that the bandage is off, consider asking for something to help you sleep.
- Use a cushion between your legs if you are a side sleeper. An airline neck pillow is great for this or a squishy stuffed animal.
- Use a heating pad on your hamstrings to soothe them.
- Try diclofenac ointment or some other over-the-counter (OTC) arthritis pain cream.
- Use the bike for 5–10 minutes before bed at night.
- Try a few exercises at night before bed to loosen up one last time for the day.

Adult Activities

You may also be ready to engage in more intimate activities. As your kneeling and flexibility improve, you will feel more comfortable experimenting with different positions. At first, some positions will be much more comfortable than others.

Here is a chart with suggestions on how to resume activity:

Returning to Adult Activity after Knee Replacement		
Position	Degree of Difficulty	Illustrative Example
Spooning/side-lying with the new knee up toward the ceiling	Low	
Sitting on a chair	Low/Medium	
Edge of bed—lying on the bed partially	Low/Medium	
Lying with the new knee up toward the ceiling	Medium	
Face down—on elbows, lying down with the new knee toward the mattress	High	
Kneeling	High	

After knee replacement surgery, you should only consider resuming adult activities when you feel ready. If you have questions, ask your surgeon. This isn't the time to be shy.

You can expect gradual improvement in comfort for up to a year or longer. Keep experimenting; as your range of motion improves, you will get more comfortable.

Practice will build confidence. *Smile and have fun!*

Kneeling

Yes! You can kneel on your new knee! It will take time, effort, and patience.

Here is a process to begin to kneel on your replaced knee: Six weeks after surgery is typically a good time to start desensitization. To begin, you should have 90 degrees of knee flexion.

Here are the progression levels to try. Only progress to the next level once you are comfortable at the current level (courtesy of Samantha Smith, DPT).

Level 1: Find a sturdy chair with arms to hold onto. Slowly kneel with a cushy pillow under your knee. Goal: kneel for 2-5 seconds at a time for 3 minutes. When you can do this comfortably twice a day, move to Level 2.

Level 2: Kneel on the couch or a padded chair without a pillow under your knee. Kneel for 3 minutes. Practice this twice a day. When you can do this comfortably twice a day, move to Level 3.

Level 3: Kneel on the ground with a thick cushion under your knee. Kneel for up to 5 minutes. Practice this twice a day. When you can do this comfortably twice a day, move to Level 4.

Level 4: Kneel on the ground with a pillow under your knee that is not as thick as you used in level 3. Kneel for up to 5 minutes. Practice this twice a day. When you can do this comfortably twice a day, move to Level 5.

Level 5: Kneel on the floor with a beach towel folded up under your knee for 5 minutes. Practice this twice a day. When you can comfortably do this twice a day, move to Level 6.

Level 6: Kneel on a carpeted floor without a towel. Kneel for 5 minutes. Practice this twice a day. When you can do this comfortably twice a day, move to Level 7.

Level 7: Continue to slowly increase the amount of time you are kneeling and change the surfaces from soft to hard.

During my recovery and while working on kneeling, I found the Kneely Pad incredibly helpful. I still use it today if I'm kneeling on a hard surface.

Here is a link to get 15% off your own Kneely Pad:

getkneely.com/discount/Diana15

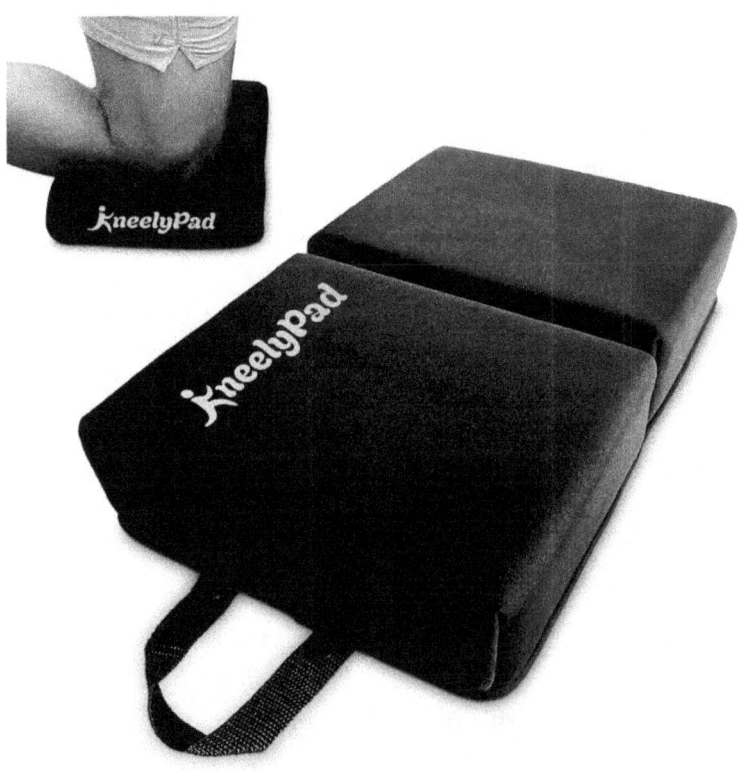

Diana's Story: Returning to Work Too Soon

During my surgery recovery, my employer was willing to be flexible and let me return to work part-time so I would have time for physical therapy.

Here was the harsh reality. It is tough to be comfortable sitting at a desk for more than an hour. I wasn't ready to be back on video. I also found it pretty shocking when people I worked with compared having a pulled shoulder muscle on the same scale as having BOTH my knees replaced as to what they thought my recovery time should be to resume travel.

I went into a mental tailspin when I learned I was suddenly taking on more work after another colleague left unexpectedly.

This is my cautionary tale about not being in a hurry to return to work. Your mindset will heavily depend on the rest you get each night. In my case, sleep was incredibly hard. I couldn't be the typical happy and positive person with my normal "No worries; you can count on me to do anything" outlook.

Keep challenging yourself to do a little—
I mean a LITTLE—more each day.

Dr. Sinha's Thoughts on Month 2 of Recovery

Remember when I said that biology is biology, and it has its own timeline? Your biology doesn't care what you think. It has zero opinion about that. In fact, it laughs at you. Remember the old saying, "Man plans; God laughs." Well, Mother Nature is the same way.

When we do this operation, we are literally cutting part of your leg off and reattaching it. It takes time to heal from that.

It takes a year to get your muscle strength back to normal, and there's nothing you can do to speed that up. That means when you start to increase your activity, like returning to work, playing a new sport, or even returning to a sport, you will have some pain, stiffness, and swelling—all normal. Eventually, that stuff will go away because, as I said, it's a year-long process for the muscles to recover and for the scar tissue to undergo its maturation process.

Your knee will be warm for about a year. That's also normal and part of the scar maturation process.

As you do things and notice that you have a little bit of an ache or a little bit of swelling, your body is telling you that, hey, it's okay for you to do this.

But you need some time to recover, so you must budget time to elevate and ice. Maybe take an anti-inflammatory medication occasionally. Eventually, you're not going to need to do that.

> I tell people this all the time. After about the first six weeks, I'm nothing more than a cheerleader. I can explain what's going to happen. I can explain what you're doing right, what you're doing wrong, when to panic, and when not to panic. I tell my patients there's no reason to panic. I will tell you when it's time for you to panic because I've seen the full range of the recovery of 10,000 different people. If you're not falling into some pattern of normality, then I will be concerned for you.

Key Takeaways for Months 1 & 2 of Recovery

1. Progress Is Not Linear
   - Recovery involves ups and downs; sometimes, you may feel like you're taking a step backward before making significant progress.
   - Celebrating small wins, like improved range of motion and walking without assistive devices, is crucial.
2. Managing Pain, Swelling, and Stiffness
   - It should become easier. Use your positive mindset to understand if you are feeling "pain" or "stiffness."
   - Weather changes do affect knee stiffness.
   - Long drives over two hours can cause swelling and stiffness.
   - Use caution if you need dental work or want a pedicure, and take antibiotics to reduce the risk of infection.

3. Returning to Physical Activity
   - Begin slowly to increase activities
   - Projects around the house
   - Adult Activities
   - Kneeling
4. Mental Exhaustion and Stress
   - Can be easily caused as you return to work or other activities
   - If you aren't getting enough rest to recover
5. For a quick reference guide of Months 1 & 2 that you can print out and easily refer to during your recovery, go to:

thekneezone.com/recoveryguides

BEND AND PROSPER

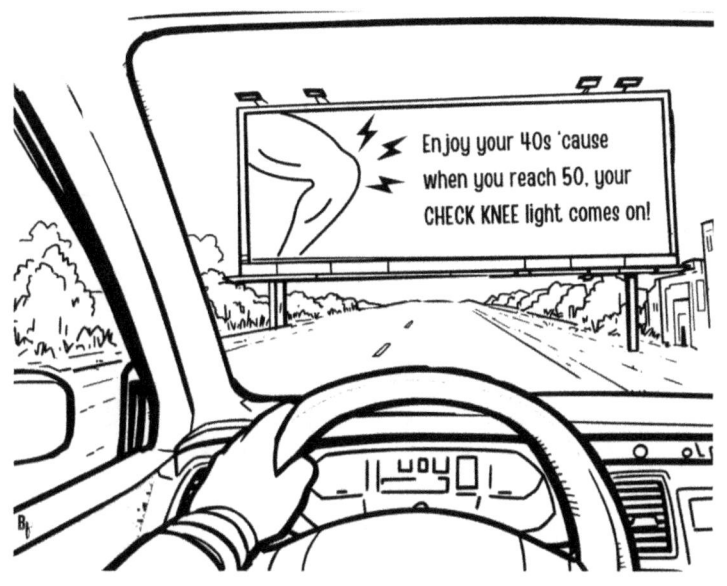

MONTH 3
GETTING BACK TO NORMAL

Happy Kneeversary! You are now three months into your bionic upgrade.

This three-month post-surgery phase is when *you* own your recovery progress going forward. It is time to remind yourself what you want to accomplish now that you have a new knee.

Are you ready to start planning bigger activities at this point in your recovery?

YES!!

Here are the things I did to ensure I was ready to "leap" into fun things again.

I rode a stationary bike for at least 15 minutes daily. Moving the pedals on the bike would loosen up stiff muscles faster than anything else, so I could start my day.

You can also use a peddler, which you can sit down in a chair and use, or lift your legs and pedal them in the air if you don't have access to a bike.

I encourage everyone to "saddle up" daily to help you with:

- Loosening up stiffness
- Building quad strength
- Improving your range of motion

You can improve your range of motion by slowly lowering your seat on an upright bike or moving closer to the pedals on a recumbent bike or peddler.

Don't let the excuse of not having a bike hold you back. You can always lie down on your back, lift your legs in the air, and pedal them.

Driving Further and Further on Your Own

I was feeling confident driving at this point. My outside solo adventures began.

I craved human interaction with a dear friend, so we planned to meet. We settled on a location about 45 miles away between our two homes.

To prepare, I followed my checklist:

1. How far would I walk, and what is the ground surface like?
2. Will there be steps to climb?
3. What is the seating arrangement at the restaurant?
4. Where would I park my car?

Thanks to Google's aerial view maps, I learned a few things from my research planning for our lunch.

- I needed to wear shoes that I could walk in easily. Based on the pictures online, the streets looked uneven.
- I decided to bring my cane to help me if needed. It is good that I did. I encountered a high curb and needed a cane for support.

- I planned where I would park my car. I wanted to park as close as possible to avoid walking too far. My incredible friend arrived early and parked right in front of the restaurant. Once I arrived, she had me take her parking spot to avoid walking too far.

Plan ahead as you venture out again; it will make things much more manageable. A little research will result in less swelling and stiffness and help you avoid overdoing it.

One week after that great lunch outing, I had the opportunity to help some family members attend an event that required driving about the same distance again. I "jumped" at the chance to leave the house again and join in some fun.

This trip was more challenging for me. I needed to walk further after parking this time. Once I arrived at the location, I realized I had forgotten my cane, as I rarely used it inside the house anymore.

It was okay not to have my cane, but I had to move slowly and carefully. Another surprise was that I had to climb a few stairs. I was grateful to have time to sit and listen to a lecture to recover. After 4,500 steps and two hours of driving that day, I was icing, elevating, and taking anti-inflammatory medicines that night to recover.

Sharing my experiences will give you ideas on what you might find challenging as you plan your outings.

Travel

I needed to travel for a meeting in my third month of recovery. This would be a solo trip and a hotel stay. This time, I was very intentional about how to manage this trip.

1. I stopped every hour of the 2 ½-hour drive to stretch. I was getting stiff pretty quickly.
2. I packed my cane, heating pad, anti-inflammatory medicines, and a plastic bag for ice.
3. I requested a hotel room near the elevator doors.
4. I also used the exercise bike at the hotel gym to relieve morning stiffness.

Tips for Traveling

1. Research the terrain ahead of time!
2. Double-check that you have the things you need:
   a. Cane/walker
   b. Plastic bag for ice on the go
   c. Anti-inflammatory medicine
   d. Heating pad
   e. Shoes you can easily walk in

This trip went very well! I logged over 9,000 steps for the first time since my knees were replaced. I drove the furthest I had driven and was prepared because I planned and double-checked that everything I needed was packed.

What does your third-month plan look like?

Dr. Sinha's Month 3 Review

Somewhere around three months or so, when I see you again, if you've reached certain milestones, I will probably say, "Okay, go forth and prosper."

You can do anything you feel comfortable doing at this point. Again, if you don't feel comfortable doing something, that's not a reason to panic. That means you're not quite ready to do that particular thing.

But if you have adequate muscle control and range of motion and reach all the milestones I'm looking for, I'll say, okay, go and try everything. You must realize that as you're doing something new, you will have a little more pain and swelling, so you must budget some time to ice and elevate to accommodate that.

All your muscles are getting used to the new knee, the new motion, the new alignment, and conditions that you haven't had for a long time. So you have to be patient.

It's relatively common for people to take an anti-inflammatory medication like ibuprofen or pain medication like acetaminophen to play a sport, whether it's golf, tennis, pickleball, exercising, or light jogging. About a third of people need that medication, even long-term. So don't panic about that. That's normal.

It's important to keep the scar covered if you're going to be in the sun. The scar can become unattractive if exposed to too much sun.

You might still feel clicking in the knee; that's normal. Eventually, that will go away as the internal scar tissue matures.

Some people struggle with bending. If they haven't reached 90 or 95 degrees of bending by three months, we might recommend a manipulation under anesthesia. That means you formed a little more scar tissue faster than expected, so we have to break it up.

The data shows that if you're going to do a manipulation, you should do it within 12 weeks of the initial surgery. If you wait longer than that, it is less effective in the long term.

In my experience, patients who need manipulations either did not take their pain medications regularly (and therefore had significant pain that prevented effective physical therapy), or overdid their exercise and physical therapy (and thus have increased pain and swelling), or worse still, didn't do any physical therapy exercise at all.

Key Takeaways for Month 3 of Recovery

1. Taking Ownership of Your Recovery
   - At three months post-surgery, you are in control of your progress.
   - Daily movement, like using a stationary bike, helps loosen stiffness, strengthen quads, and improve range of motion.
   - If you don't have a bike, alternative exercises like air pedaling can be effective.

2. Planning for Outings
   - Driving and venturing out alone becomes more manageable with careful planning.
   - Research parking, walking distances, seating, and terrain in advance to avoid unnecessary strain.
   - Bringing a cane for support can be helpful, even if you don't always need it.
3. Travel Strategies
   - Long trips require intentional preparation.
   - Stop frequently to stretch.
   - Packing essentials like ice packs, anti-inflammatory medication, and heating pads can make traveling smoother and more comfortable.
4. Adjusting to Your New Knee (Bionic Upgrade)
   - As muscles adapt to new motion and alignment, occasional pain, swelling, or clicking in the knee is normal.
   - Continuing to ice, elevate, and take anti-inflammatory medications as needed will help manage discomfort.
   - By month three, most people should reach 90–95 degrees of bending. If stiffness persists due to excessive scar tissue, a manipulation under anesthesia might be necessary within 12 weeks for the best long-term outcome.
   - Regular and balanced physical therapy is crucial for avoiding this intervention.

5. For a quick reference guide of Month 3 in your recovery, go to:

thekneezone.com/recoveryguides

MIDWAY MILESTONES

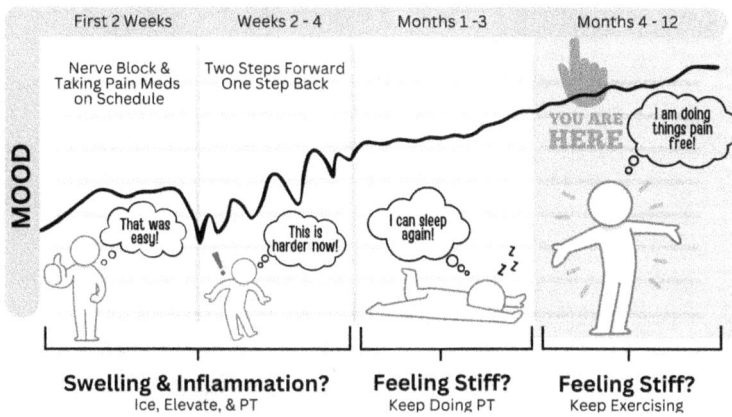

MONTHS 4 & 5
YOU'RE HALFWAY TO TOTAL HEALING!

Happy Kneeversary! You are four months into your bionic upgrade, and the good news is you are at the HALFWAY point of your recovery—based on most people.

Here are vital things you should continue to monitor as you enter Month 4:

1. Don't risk losing range of motion—yes, this can happen!
2. Keep massaging that scar to break up the scar tissue.
3. Increase the resistance and duration of your exercise bike. You can also lower the seat for a greater range of motion (ROM).
4. Now is a great time for pool therapy. If you don't have a pool, find an indoor pool in your community to use. Many cities have public-use shallow pools with easy access for this very purpose.
5. Master kneeling on a pillow. I'm a fan of the Kneely Pad, which I started using when I returned to Pilates. I'm still using it today for certain activities.
6. Stiffness/swelling/soreness/tightness—yep, this is when you need to watch what you are doing and slowly build up your activity level if you have a setback.

7. If your new knee still feels "hot," that is normal. Your body and the new bionic upgrade are still getting to know each other.
8. Challenge yourself—stairs, balancing, squats, lunges, and anything else you want to try.

Months 4 & 5 are when your recovery progresses to a point where you might forget your knee was replaced.

Day-to-day life is starting to feel pretty good—dare I say normal—most days. Fear not if you aren't quite there yet.

For most people, the time between four and six months is when you enter the zone of feeling "normal" again.

This phase of your recovery also begins a transition to tweaking your methods of managing any discomfort—remember to try to label it as "stiffness" rather than pain.

Since I had both knees replaced at the same time, my recovery was a bit more challenging. Throughout the first six months, I still experienced daily stiffness. I pedaled on my stationary bike for at least 15 minutes each morning to loosen up before doing anything else.

Starting my day on the bike would loosen me up faster than anything else I tried.

I encourage everyone to "saddle up" on a bike daily to help you with:

- Loosening up stiffness
- Building quad strength
- Improving your range of motion

Months 4 & 5 are significant points in your recovery to begin returning to activities you may be missing out on. For me, that was getting back on the golf course. It was challenging on the uneven terrain, but it felt great to be back on the course, and I reminded myself that it would only get better with every outing.

Ease into activities and sports slowly. Plan to shorten the time of the activity and build up to more time as you feel comfortable and pain-free.

If you feel ready, it is probably time for you to try light activities again, such as:

- Tennis
- Pickleball
- Golf
- Biking outside
- Walking further than you have been
- Gentle hikes

What is it you've been looking forward to doing?

Are you ready to start planning bigger activities at this point in your recovery?

It's possible you'll end up doing too much, which can cause you to feel tired and sore. When this happens, take a break immediately to ice and elevate. A heating pad may also be helpful. Either ice or heat is acceptable in Months 4 & 5.

Start slow and give yourself grace as you take on more.

Swimming Pool Physical Therapy

If you are interested in pool exercises, here are some I used during my recovery.

Doing "too much" in the pool is easier than you think. Please limit your physical therapy pool activity and slowly increase the time you spend on it.

Fifteen minutes in the pool the first time is enough to move the needle. Increase the time spent on exercises in the pool gradually.

Set a timer, and don't overdo it.

Simple exercises for the pool:

1. Walk forward and backward to warm up for 5-10 minutes.
2. Find a step to do lunges using your new knee.
3. Squats in the pool—hold on to the pool's edge in the shallow end.
4. Improve leg extension by raising your bionic leg on a wall and holding it straight.
5. Use a pool noodle to bicycle your legs in the pool. Ride the noodle.
6. Sit on the pool stairs and practice standing up and sitting down.

Be sure to limit yourself to no more than 30 minutes in the pool doing exercises. Although moving in the pool feels so easy, you can easily do too much and will feel stiff without that extraordinary buoyancy outside the pool.

Be sure to protect your scar with waterproof sunscreen for the first 12 months!

Dr. Sinha's Important Milestones

Remember that I mentioned certain milestones after surgery?

The first milestone after knee replacement is full extension, or a knee that straightens completely. We want you to achieve that within the first two weeks. If you don't achieve it at the end of two weeks, you can still achieve it, so there's no reason to panic. Your leg with your new knee will be fully straightened out during your surgery, and if you can keep or regain full extension early on, your overall recovery will go much faster.

The second milestone is 90 degrees of bending. There's a rule of thumb that how much bending you get after the knee replacement parallels what you had going into the knee replacement. I don't entirely agree with that because a lot of it has to do with pain management and what the surgeon does in surgery. I published a paper about 20 years ago that showed that with the techniques I use, patients actually achieved about 130 degrees of flexion at final recovery, even if they had restricted flexion prior to surgery.

So again, the milestone at three months is to bend to at least 90 degrees. If you're not at 90 degrees, that's concerning. But if you're at 95 degrees, that's not necessarily concerning because you will gradually get more range of motion up to one year from surgery. Typically, compared to where you are at three months, you can expect another 15 to 20 degrees at 12 months. So don't get worked up about bending until the three-month point.

> Strength is significant. It's not likely that you'll lose range of motion after three months, but if you don't regain your strength, you can still develop muscle pain as you return to being active. You don't have to exercise or do three sets of exercises every day, but if you can exercise every other day at this point, that's what I'm looking for.

Key Takeaways for Month 4 of Recovery

1. Protect Your Range of Motion (ROM)
   - Continue working on flexibility to prevent loss of motion.
   - Lowering your bike seat can help improve ROM.
   - Pool Therapy can also be very therapeutic and help with range of motion.
2. Scar Care
   - Massage Matters. Keep massaging your scar to break up scar tissue and improve mobility.
   - Scar strips are helpful for sun protection.
3. Increase Activity & Resistance
   - Gradually build endurance by using an exercise bike.
   - Try pool therapy.
   - Challenge yourself with stairs, squats, and lunges.
   - Consider returning to sports you miss playing.
4. Manage Stiffness & Swelling
   - Monitor soreness and tightness.
   - Adjust activity levels to avoid setbacks.

- If your knee still feels "hot," that's normal.
- If you still hear clicking in your new knee, that's also normal.

5. Work on kneeling to ease back into it and other movements.

For a quick reference guide of Months 4 & 5 that you can print out and refer to during your recovery, go to:

thekneezone.com/recoveryguides

MONTH 6 & BEYOND
THE HOMESTRETCH

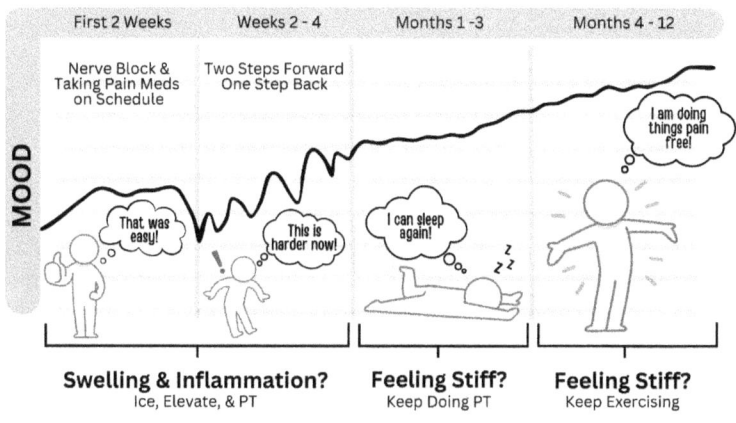

START SAYING "YES!"

Queue the music, and get on your party hat. You have entered Month 6!

Happy Kneeversary!

Here are vital things you should continue to monitor as you enter Month 6:

1. Quads still need strengthening—this is not the point at which to stop. Challenge yourself to exercise every other day, even two minutes of climbing stairs, balancing, squats, lunges, and anything else you want to try.
2. Are you ready to up your game with walking, working out, traveling, and anything else you might be passionate about? Now is the time to push yourself if you have been holding back.
3. Keep massaging the scar to break up the scar tissue, and decide if you still need to use scar prevention creams.
4. Are you feeling stiff? Hit the bike—it will likely be your friend for a while.
5. Conquer the stairs once and for all—if you haven't yet.
6. Stiffness/swelling/soreness/tightness—yep, this is when you need to watch what you are doing and slowly build up your activity level if you have a setback.

It is time to move forward boldly, try everything you said "no" to just six months ago, and get back to living your life.

Like life, you'll have great days and enjoy activities fully without pain. You might have other days that leave you feeling stiff and disappointed.

> ### Diana's Story: Mastering Stairs
>
>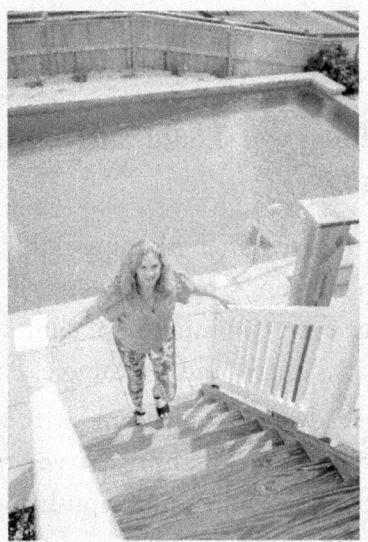
>
> *On a day in Month 11 of my recovery, I climbed 23 flights of stairs and was sore. Feeling sore should not have been a shock; instead, I used a hot tub and celebrated doing something I couldn't have done before my surgery.*
>
> *There is no way I could have walked up and down 23 flights of stairs before my knee replacements without being in tremendous pain. How you perceive your progress is really important.*

I'm still pushing myself to do more and not let my perception of what I can and can't do hold me back. This shift in my perception includes exercise, adult activities, kneeling on the floor, and anything else I think I might not be ready to "try yet"—pickleball might be next on that list.

You may also find that your other leg hurts at this point in your recovery. After all, you put lots of extra weight on it in the last few months and probably years' worth before you had your knee replaced. If you have osteoarthritis, it is not limited to one body joint.

Treat that other leg with some TLC: a heating pad, massage, and some of those physical therapy exercises you did at the beginning of your recovery. If this doesn't relieve your pain, you might want to see your surgeon and have them decide if you should have that knee examined and X-rayed to understand the severity of the arthritis condition.

I hope you will celebrate your monthly "Kneeversary" and your good fortune of fully recovering and being part of a bionic community.

> **What Dr. Sinha Says to Expect Beyond 6 Months**
>
> If everything has gone well, I usually remove all restrictions at the three-month point. You will continue to recover for up to one year after surgery. In some cases, like revision surgeries, it takes up to two years.
>
> I've seen people do extraordinary things after knee replacement: I have a patient who is a national champion powerlifter, another plays on a national champion over-55 volleyball

team, others heli-ski (jump out of a helicopter to ski down a mountain), surf, race bicycles, and play basketball, golf, tennis, and pickleball. I even have a marathoner who has run two marathons after his surgery.

Some surgeons recommend against impact activities. However, having spent many years studying the biomechanics of knees, my feeling is that a well-functioning knee can withstand these high-impact sports.

What will you be able to do after your knee replacement? I want to say whatever you want, but that's not exactly true. Even though I will let you do whatever you can, you will find that some activities are more comfortable than others and, therefore, more enjoyable for you. And what you can do in one year will be different than in six months. You just have to experiment and figure out what you can do and have fun doing it.

Key Takeaways for Month 6 of Knee Replacement Recovery

1. Keep Strengthening Your Quads
    - Don't stop now!
    - Continue challenging yourself with stairs, squats, lunges, and other exercises every other day.
2. Push Your Limits & Say "YES"
    - Now is the time to embrace walking, traveling, and other activities you may have avoided.
    - Shift your mindset and explore new possibilities.

3. Manage Stiffness & Recovery
   - Use the exercise bike.
   - Massage your scar.
   - Be mindful of soreness.
   - If your other leg is hurting, give it some TLC with heat, massage, and early rehab exercises.
4. Celebrate Your Progress
   - Perception is key.
   - Some days will be great, and others may bring stiffness.
   - Acknowledge how far you've come—small wins matter!
5. The Future Is Bright
   - Full recovery can take up to a year (or more for revisions).
   - People have gone on to do amazing things, from powerlifting to marathons.
   - Keep experimenting and find what works for you!

For a quick reference guide of Month 6 that you can print out and refer to during your recovery, go to:

thekneezone.com/recoveryguides

KICKING THE CAN DOWN THE ROAD

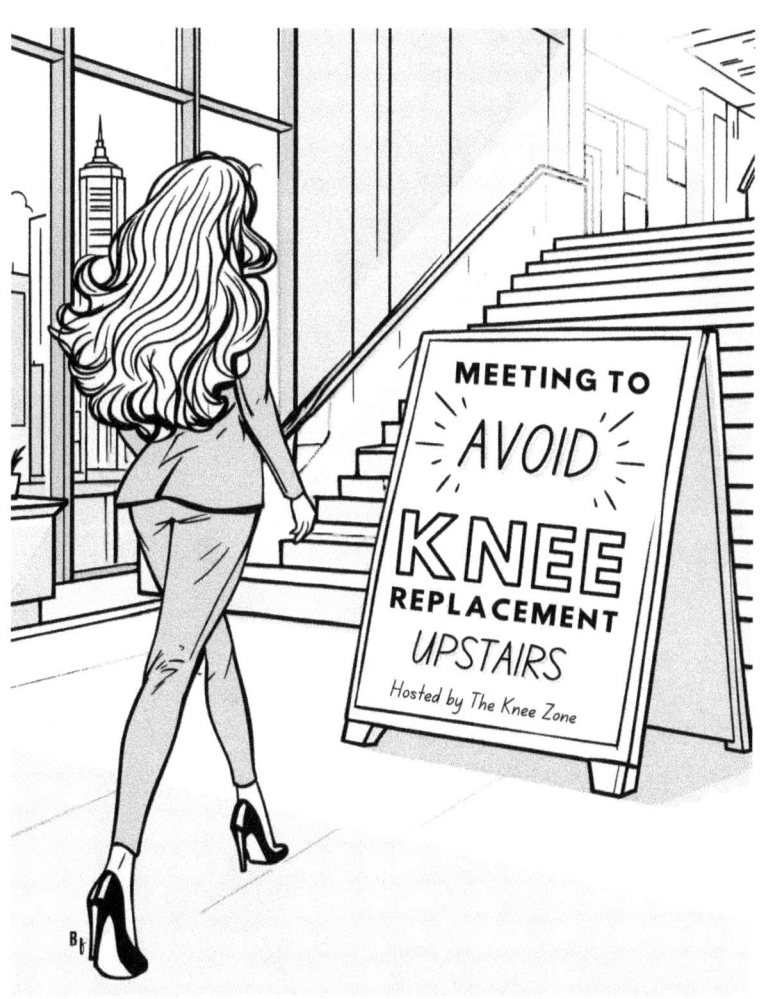

TIPS ON HOW TO AVOID SURGERY

If you jumped ahead to this section, chances are you're not quite ready to contemplate surgery or read the rest of this book. That was me until I had stabbing pain in both my knees, abruptly waking me up at night.

I made it my mission to try everything possible to keep working, traveling, golfing, wearing high heels, and avoiding surgery.

I was able to try many things to help postpone my surgery for a long time.

Below are the things I did and a brief description of each. These don't need to be tried one at a time, in sequential order, and many can be combined.

The options I tried allowed me to postpone knee replacement surgery for eight years. I was diagnosed with osteoarthritis (OA), which eventually progressed to painful bone-on-bone arthritis in both knees. Maybe a few of these can help you "kick the can down the road" until you're ready for surgery.

1. Physical therapy
2. Cortisone injections
3. Gel injections
4. Platelet-rich plasma injections
5. Stem cell injections

6. Apos shoe therapy
7. Kinesiology tape
8. Weight management
9. Pain medicine
10. Rest, ice, and elevate
11. Supplements
12. Laser treatments
13. Arthritis knee brace
14. Ambulatory aid devices

Physical Therapy

- Physical therapy strengthens muscles, taking pressure off the damaged bone and cartilage.
- It improves flexibility, which may improve the health of the remaining cartilage.
- A physical therapist will create a personalized treatment plan for you.
- You'll learn exercises, stretches, and manual techniques to practice at home.
- Your physical therapist can use various pain relief methods such as ultrasound, electrical stimulation, massage, and red light therapy.

Cortisone Injections

- Cortisone injections can provide significant pain relief from arthritis, tendonitis, or bursitis.
- May reduce inflammation, swelling, and associated discomfort.
- Can improve mobility.

- Are a common nonsurgical option.
- Are quick and convenient with minimal downtime.
- Often provide pain relief shortly after the injection.
- Can be repeated usually in three-month intervals.
- May interact with some diseases and medications.
- Typically provide relief for up to three months and may be covered by insurance.

Gel Injections

Gel injections, also known as viscosupplementation, use hyaluronic acid to lubricate the joint, cushion the bones, and relieve pain.

- Gel injections can improve joint function by increasing the viscosity of the synovial fluid in the knee joint.
- Generally produces minimal side effects for repeated use over time. May be repeated often.
- Non-Systemic Treatment: Gel injections directly target the affected joint, delivering the gel precisely where it's needed without affecting the rest of the body.
- Insurance may cover injections every six months.

Platelet-Rich Plasma Injections

Platelet-rich plasma (PRP) is derived from your blood.

- Platelet-rich plasma injections can provide significant pain relief from arthritis, tendonitis, or bursitis.
- May reduce inflammation, swelling, and associated discomfort.
- Might improve mobility by alleviating pain and inflammation.
- Quick and convenient with minimal downtime.

- Many people experience pain relief shortly after the injection.
- If this option works for you, PRP can be repeated as often as you wish.
- Typically not covered by insurance.

Stem Cell Injections

- Stem cell injections can provide long-lasting pain relief for osteoarthritis, tendonitis, and bursitis.
- For those who find it effective, it could last over a year.
- Options include using:
  - Fat-derived cells
  - Bone marrow-derived cells
- Stimulates the body's cells to decrease inflammation.
- Does not regrow cartilage.
- Typically not covered by insurance and can be very expensive.

Apos Shoe Therapy

Apos is a noninvasive medical device that is personalized to treat your pain by retraining your gait (how you walk) to help you move and live better.

- Special shoes with custom pods (aka pertupods) adjust throughout your therapy journey.
- Along with physical therapy, these shoes can adjust how you walk to offload the damaged joint.
- They may also help with lower back pain.
- Apos may be covered by insurance.

Kinesiology Tape (KT)

- Kinesiology tape offers extra support to muscles and joints.
- Can help some people protect their range of motion and reduce pain for those with knee arthritis.
- Creates support by balancing the muscles on the knee and relieving pressure on the kneecap and its tendon.
- Can be used daily for an unlimited amount of time.
- Can easily be applied by yourself by watching a YouTube video or asking a physical therapist to show you how.
- Can be purchased online or in drugstores.

Weight Management

- Weight loss can reduce your knee pain.
- With every step, your knee takes on three to seven times your total weight and five to ten times with stairs.
- Shedding 10 pounds takes 30–70 pounds of pressure off your knees.
- A lighter "you" eases pressure on your joints, reduces inflammation, and helps you get around more easily.

Pain Medicine

Discuss any pain medicine with your doctor before taking it to ensure it will not interfere with other medications or health conditions.

- The best option for arthritis pain is a combination of Tylenol (Acetaminophen) and anti-inflammatory medications.

- Common over-the-counter anti-inflammatory options include:
  ○ Advil/Motrin (Ibuprofen)
  ○ Aleve (Naproxen)
- Prescription anti-inflammatory medications include:
  ○ Celebrex (Celecoxib)
  ○ Mobic (Meloxicam)
  ○ Naproxen and ibuprofen are also available in prescription strengths
  ○ Voltaren arthritis gel and/or pills (Diclofenac)

Rest, Ice, and Elevate

- Ice can be your best friend as you continue to avoid surgery.
- Keep an empty gallon plastic bag handy to fill with ice on the go to help you if you're having a rough day.
- Elevating your leg will help reduce swelling.
- Ideally, elevate your toes above the level of your nose.
- Apply an ice pack for 15-20 minutes after any exercise.

Supplements

Supplements might help:

- Decrease inflammation
- Decrease pain
- Slow down cartilage breakdown
- Improve muscle strength
- Improve health
- Prevent disease

The quality of the supplements makes a difference.

Laser Therapy

Laser therapy works by penetrating deep into the knee joint tissues, where it can:

- Stimulate new cell growth
- Increase oxygen and nutrient flow, which can trigger endorphins
- Help the immune system heal tissue and build connective tissue
- Open blood vessels to reduce swelling

Low-level laser therapy (LLLT) is used to treat osteoarthritis (OA).

LLLT beams light energy into the knee in 30-second pulses without damaging skin tissue.

Studies have shown that LLLT can significantly improve pain, knee function, and walking distance compared to no treatment.

Insurance and Medicare may cover LLLT.

Arthritis Knee Brace

When knees become deformed from arthritis, they often become crooked. An unloader brace can shift some of the weight from the bad side of your knee to the good side. This accomplishes the following:

- Provides stability to the knee
- Decreases pressure on the more damaged side
- Decreases inflammatory chemicals from being produced in the knee

The most effective knee braces have to be prescribed by a doctor. You can experiment with non-prescription, but a poorly fitting brace can cause other problems.

Ambulatory Aid Devices

These include canes, crutches, and walkers. The idea is to offload pressure on the damaged knee. The benefits are:

- Using a cane on the opposite hand from your arthritic knee takes 50% of your body weight off that knee
- A single crutch will provide the same benefits as a cane
- Using a walker can take up to 75% of your body weight off the damaged knee and give you added support when walking

Please ensure you are properly fitted and instructed in their safe usage.

> ### Dr. Sinha's Thoughts on Kicking the Can Down the Road
>
> The primary reason we do knee replacement surgery is because of arthritis pain. It's sad but true: arthritis happens in the best of families. What's really frustrating for somebody who treats arthritis is the nonchalant attitude many healthcare providers have about it.
>
> How often do you hear—even from your doctors—"Oh, it's just arthritis. What are you going to do?" Well, as somebody who treats arthritis, there's a lot you can do to slow

it down. You can't stop it. It will continue to progress. It worsens in 100 percent of cases, but you can slow the progression.

Muscle strength and flexibility are two things that help improve the nutrition of the cartilage that's being damaged from arthritis. So the more you can do to work on muscle strength and flexibility, the slower the cartilage will wear away.

You can't do weight training in many cases because it hurts too much, but things like Pilates or yoga also build muscle strength and especially flexibility, so they're very important to try.

Keeping your weight down is also essential. Every 10 pounds you gain adds up to 70 pounds of pressure on your knee. Conversely, every 10 pounds you lose takes up to 70 pounds of pressure off your knee.

I've had patients lose 10 or 20 pounds before surgery to reduce their surgery risks, and they've actually come back to me and said, "My knee feels so good. I don't think I need the surgery right now."

Once again, you're not going to stop the arthritis from progressing, but you can slow down the progression.

Bracing helps with stability but can cause the muscles to weaken because you're not using them to maintain stability. So, bracing is something to use with caution.

However, there is a type of brace called an unloader brace, which specifically pushes the knee joint in the opposite direction of the arthritis. It allows you to shift the weight from the damaged part of the knee to the less damaged part.

By shifting the weight, you take about 40 to 60 percent of the pressure off the damaged part of the knee. Less pressure means less pain. Those braces work best if you start them early in the arthritis disease.

When your primary care physician says, "Oh, well, it's arthritis. What are you going to do?" think, "Unloader brace, flexibility, and strength. That's what I'm going to do because it will slow down the progression of arthritis."

Medications don't slow down the arthritis progression. Things like acetaminophen and anti-inflammatory medications help block the pain by decreasing inflammation and blocking some pain receptors at the site of the damaged arthritic knee.

If you get to the point where you need opioids, you're ready for surgery. In fact, you should have already had surgery by that point because the research data shows that opioids don't improve function in an arthritic knee.

Other treatment modalities to address the pain, but not prevent or reverse the arthritis, are injectables. We can inject corticosteroids into the knee that help to block the pain receptors and decrease the inflammation.

We can inject ketorolac (trade name Toradol) into the knee, which does the same.

We can inject viscosupplementation or hyaluronic acid, which is a gel material. It's the same molecule that your joint fluid is made out of. Technically, it's considered a device. When injected into the knee, it coats the surfaces of the bone, decreases some of the friction in the damaged knee, and also causes the production of a protein called lubricin, which helps to reduce the friction in the knee.

Those injections help to decrease the pain as well.

In the last 15 or 20 years, a lot of work has been done on biological materials like platelet-rich plasma (PRP) or stem cells, and there are various stem cell preparations out there.

The long and the short of it is that those things do not regrow much, if any, cartilage. Less-than-scrupulous companies promote cartilage regrowth, but no studies have actually shown significant enough cartilage growth to suggest that it's reversing arthritis.

But like the other injectables, they help decrease pain by various biological mechanisms, shutting off inflammation and blocking pain receptors from firing.

In terms of stem cells, you can use fat-derived stem cells or bone marrow-derived stem cells. Those all appear to have about the same degree of efficacy. In younger patients, the bone marrow seems to be slightly better than the fat. Again, this data is not 100 percent clear-cut and continues to evolve.

Lastly, preparations that claim to take tissue or stem cells from the placenta or Wharton's jelly from newborns have not been shown to give significant sustained pain relief. Plus, they're not FDA-approved or regulated by the FDA, so beware of their use. Usually, though, they are safe but can be quite expensive.

Oral supplementation may have some value in decreasing inflammation in general in your body. There's been a push in the last half-decade to have patients take more supplements going into surgery to build up their tissues, not so much to decrease arthritis but to make their healing better.

The basic story behind any supplement is that you want to increase the antioxidants in your body to help healing. However, you also don't want to use supplements that have compounds that thin your blood because that just causes more bleeding and bruising at the time of surgery, and the bruising can cause pain.

Many insurance companies require patients to try physical therapy before knee replacement surgery. The premise is that some people have arthritis-related pain, like various bursitis-type conditions. If you can eliminate those things or at least decrease them, then the pain is lessened.

Similarly, physical therapy can increase strength for some patients to the point where they have less pain in the knee. In my experience, if you have end-stage arthritis, physical therapy does not help, despite what some insurance companies claim. Again, they look at research papers that have been debunked, but they still have them in their databases as the primary guideline.

But if you have early arthritis, physical therapy can be very beneficial.

> There's been recent conversation about red light therapy, which increases the production of an enzyme in the cellular mitochondria (boy, that's a mouthful!). The benefit of that is to reduce inflammation by stimulating various cellular processes.
>
> I have used musculoskeletal dual-wavelength lasers in the past. The concept is to increase blood flow and stimulate some DNA upregulation. Again, I don't think it reverses arthritis, but it can help with some of the pain associated with arthritis, particularly soft tissue pain.

Key Takeaways on Tips to Avoid Knee Replacement Surgery

1. These are options you can investigate and do on your own:
   - Weight management
   - Rest, ice, and elevate
   - Supplements
   - KT tape
2. Injection options to consider:
   - Cortisone injections
   - Gel injections
   - Platelet Rich Plasma injections
   - Stem cell injections

3. Additional options to seek from care providers:
   - Physical therapy
   - Apos shoe therapy
   - Laser therapy
   - Unloader brace

What If I'm Still in Pain After Trying Options?

If you reach a point where you can no longer do the things you love without the distraction of pain, you are probably ready for knee replacement surgery.

Due to medical, physical, and financial requirements, not everyone has the same options I tried along the way.

If you are out of options, it is time to return to the beginning of the book and read the chapter titled: "Is Putting It Off Putting You at Risk?"

FINAL THOUGHTS

Diana's Final Thoughts

When I set out to write this book with my husband, my goal was to create something informative, easy to understand, and valuable for anyone considering or recovering from a knee replacement.

By sharing my personal experience after having both my knees replaced—along with insights from a knee replacement surgeon—I wanted to provide information that wasn't readily available to patients.

I hope you found it helpful and will pass it along to someone who would benefit from what they "knee'd" to know.

Before we go, here are some final thoughts from Dr. Sinha on the history and future of knee replacement surgery …

Dr. Sinha Shares the History—and Future—of Knee Replacement Surgery

Knee replacement has come a long way in the five decades since it became a common procedure. In the first decade of knee replacement design (1970-1980), over 100 different implant versions were developed.

Although surgeons and engineers had a reasonably good understanding of normal knee biomechanics, manufacturing limitations and immature materials science prevented them from effectively replicating nature's design. They had to accept certain constraints, leading to numerous design concepts. Nevertheless, knee replacement proved to be a safe and effective solution for older patients with severe and debilitating arthritis.

Encouraged by early success in elderly patients, surgeons began performing knee replacements in younger, more active individuals. These patients put greater demands on the implants, exposing significant limitations in both manufacturing and surgical techniques. Among the issues that emerged:

- Early plastic wear and breakage
- Knee replacement instability
- Residual pain and stiffness
- Poor flexibility
- Inability to return to sports

Researchers then spent the next three decades engineering solutions to these problems. By around 1995, when I began practicing, several key principles had become widely accepted:

- Accurate bone cuts were critical for proper leg alignment.
- Bone cement was the most durable method for securing implants.
- Ligament balancing techniques were essential for stability.
- Certain designs supported higher activity levels.
- Sterilization methods impacted plastic durability.
- A broader range of implant sizes gave surgeons more intraoperative flexibility.
- Women's knees differed from men's.

Despite these advances, 10 to 20% of patients remained unhappy with knee replacements. Their most common complaints included:

- Residual pain
- Stiffness
- Limited flexibility
- Long recovery time
- Lack of natural movement
- Insufficient stability for sports

To address these concerns, several new technologies emerged in the early 21st century, including:

- Implant design innovations:
  o High-flexion knees (allowing up to 155 degrees of bend)
  o Gender-specific implants (male vs. female shapes)
  o Single-radius femoral components
- Advancements in surgical techniques and tools:
  o Computer navigation (GPS for the operating room)
  o Patient-specific cutting guides
  o Minimally invasive instruments
  o Quad-sparing surgical incisions
  o Robotic-assisted surgery

I was involved in many innovations, from early robotic adoption to designing new implants and refining surgical techniques.

Yet, after nearly 15 years of "innovation," the dissatisfaction rate remained at 10% to 20%. Research comparing different implant designs and surgical techniques—robotic vs. non-robotic, for example—showed little difference in patient outcomes.

At the same time, significant progress was made in understanding pain management, which has been just as crucial as implant design for improving recovery. Modern pain control strategies now include:

- Preoperative pain medications

- Nerve blocks
- Increased use of anti-inflammatories and steroids over opioids
- Regular dosing rather than on-demand pain relief (preventing pain is more effective than treating it)

Meanwhile, deregulated medical advertising allowed companies, hospitals, and surgeons to make exaggerated and sometimes misleading claims about the superiority of certain implants or techniques. As a result, everyone you talk to seems to have their personal favorite—whether it's robotics, navigation, or custom implants.

One of my mentors, Dr. Richard Rothman, used to say, "Good surgeons have good results." He was right. A good surgeon possesses knowledge, technical skill, and wisdom. Above all, choosing the right surgeon is the most important decision you can make. That requires more than just trusting your primary care physician—you need to do your research. Fortunately, today's data is readily available across multiple platforms.

The philosopher Voltaire once said, "Politicians use statistics much like a drunk uses a lamppost—more for support than illumination." My mentor, Dr. Robert Booth, adapted this to orthopedics: "Surgeons use the literature much like a drunk uses a lamppost—more for support than illumination."

He warned us to be wary of those who selectively (mis) quote research to support their biases. Meta-analyses—large studies combining multiple research papers—suggest that most so-called advances make little long-term difference. These tools, like hammers, work well when used correctly, but they are not magic solutions.

This brings me back to the most important takeaway:

1. **Choose a good surgeon.**
2. **Let them do what they do best.**
3. **Follow their instructions.**

That is your best path to a successful outcome.

The Next Breakthrough in Knee Replacement: Customization

As mentioned, 10 to 20% of patients remain unhappy after knee replacement, despite various techniques and technologies we've tried. I've personally tested most of them.

The conclusion was clear: the implants themselves were the limiting factor. Despite design innovations, we never truly matched patient anatomy, and the fundamental shape of the implant remained unchanged. Essentially, Willie Shoemaker, the 4'11" horse jockey, and Wilt Chamberlain, the 7'1" basketball player, would have received the same implant design. Intuitively, that doesn't make sense—they are entirely different people.

With any given implant brand, there might be 10 sizes, but the smallest and largest shared the same shape, as if Willie and Wilt had identical knee anatomy. Likewise, right knee implants were simply mirror images of left knee implants.

This design approach stemmed from using population averages rather than individual anatomy.

When Diana received her custom implants, she immediately noticed that her right knee had a different shape and size than her left—something traditional implants overlook. (Check out thekneezone.com/education for a video explaining these differences.)

Around 2009, Conformis (now restor3d) introduced a game-changing manufacturing technique that allowed for the rapid and cost-effective production of patient-specific implants. This marked the next evolution of total knee replacement—customization. I was fortunate to join the surgeon design team during this breakthrough.

Today, we can create implants tailored to each patient's unique knee shape and size. Even the surgical tools are custom-made, snapping onto the patient's bone for precise alignment, ensuring accurate bone removal and implant placement.

In most cases, a customized knee replacement doesn't cost extra. Research—now spanning over 100 studies and 150,000 procedures worldwide—demonstrates that personalized knee implants:

- Have a lower infection rate
- Feel more like a natural knee
- Are preferred 7-to-1 over off-the-shelf implants by patients who've had both
- Have a lower reoperation rate for all causes

For these reasons, I recommend custom implants for most patients. However, some individuals with severe deformities or unstable ligaments may not yet qualify. Those solutions are coming, but we're not quite there yet.

I acknowledge my potential bias in favor of custom implants. In my opinion, they're the best option for most patients. While 80-90% of patients are satisfied with standard knee implants, custom knee implants have pushed satisfaction rates to 93-97%, reducing the unhappy group to just 3-7%.

Will we ever reach 99-100%? My molecular biology background tells me not with metal and plastic—biological solutions are still decades away.

LET'S KEEP IN TOUCH!

We are here to help you on your journey beyond the pages of this book.

As we actively look for new ways to help you avoid, prepare for, and recover from knee replacement surgery, we invite you to join our online community and speak to us directly.

You can learn more about what we offer by visiting:

TheKneeZone.com

Connect with us on Facebook here:

facebook.com/TheKneeZonePage

Find us on Instagram (where we "try" to post fun things):

instagram.com/the_knee_zone

For educational videos on YouTube and to see Diana share her story, visit:

youtube.com/@TheKneeZone

If you would like 1-on-1 coaching directly or are interested in joining a coaching group to help you with your journey, head over to:

thekneezone.com/services

Reach out and let us know how you're doing!

ACKNOWLEDGMENTS

Thank you ... from Diana

For my coaching clients, who provided me with the nudge to publish a book.

For my friends and family who cheered me on when I decided to embark on an entrepreneurial journey.

For my 90-Day Elite Group and special Beach Bosses who constantly encouraged me to bring my gift to the world. You are **all** really pretty!

And for my husband, Raj—he encouraged me in my postoperative nerve block haze when I had the idea to create The Knee Zone.

I'm energized by people on their own "bionic" upgrade journey, and I look forward to helping you on yours.

Coaching clients: Chrysteen B., Kathryn B., Heather C., Lisa C., AJ D., Elizabeth F., Todd H., Janet K., John K., Jean M., and Peggy M., Mark W. for helping us test and confirm all the content and suggestions we shared.

Dr Kipling Sharpe and the OrthoArizona team for performing Diana's bilateral knee replacements.

Vangie Weems, amazing physician's assistant to Dr. Sinha.

Conformis/restor3d team for creating a second set of my custom knee replacements to show to people.

Brian and Mary, thank you for having a fantastic home available for my post-op recovery.

Mieko, thank you for sharing Caring Bridge, outstanding final proofreading, and cheering me on and making me laugh until we cried during the graphics research phase.

Janis and Wendy for their regular check-ins after my surgery and telling me funny things when I needed a break from reality.

Vicki, for making my first solo outing a success.

Danielle, for surviving Italy with me.

Megan, Ryann, and Rebecca at Club Pilates, Temple.

Bill, Sarah, and Kim at Stretch Lab, Temple.

Allison, my physical therapist in Arizona at OrthoArizona

My physical therapy team at Integrity Rehab in Texas: Laura, Kylie, Holly, and front desk friend Wyatt.

Larry, Rabindra, and Nirmala, thank you for driving me to physical therapy for the first few weeks after my surgery.

Ava, Sid, YoYo, Kayla, and Hunter for being the best Santa's helpers when I couldn't get off the sofa to help decorate right after my surgery. You were truly Christmas miracles.

Lori Lynn (architect/editor/coach) for guiding me step-by-step on how to write, edit, refine, and bring a book into the world.

Shanda Trofe (design/launch), Mary Rembert (editing/proofreading), Lora Campbell—Your Brand Fashionista (illustrator), and Leremy Stick Figures (adult cartoons).

Chrysteen Braun and Janet Kaiser—brave first draft manuscript readers and The Knee Zone coaching clients—my Bionic Beauties.

Our professional colleague reviewers: Nicholas Abidi, M.D., FAAOS; Yana Cheatham, PT DPT; Jon Elbert, PT DPT; Lara Herzog, PT DPT; and Kipling Sharpe, M.D., FAAOS.

Our beta readers: AJ D., Amy S., Bonnie S., Brenda V., Charlyn R., Dave L., Jean M., Julia C., Kate A., Kathryn B., Kati J., Lisa C., Lora C., Mieko O., Peggy M., Sheila J., and Yari M.

Last but not least, my fantastic husband convinced me to stop living in pain and replace my knees after years of debate. You were right, Raj. I should have done it sooner.

—**Diana Braun, CHPC**

Thank you ... from Raj

I would like to express my deepest gratitude to the following people:

My astounding wife, best friend, and co-author Diana, for giving me a forum to teach a plurality of patients about knee replacement, rather than the way I have been doing it for decades—one patient at a time; for tolerating football widowhood every year; and for enriching my life in ways I never could have imagined.

My surgical teachers and mentors: Dr. Richard Rothman, Dr. Lawrence Crossett, Dr. Harry Rubash, Dr. Robert Booth, and Dr. William Hozack—giants in our industry who conveyed their knowledge and expertise to a multitude of surgical students, including me.

The over 10,000 surgical patients who trusted me to try to better their lives.

The over one million patients who currently have a hip or knee replacement implant that I helped design.

—Raj Sinha, MD, PhD, FAAOS

ABOUT THE AUTHORS

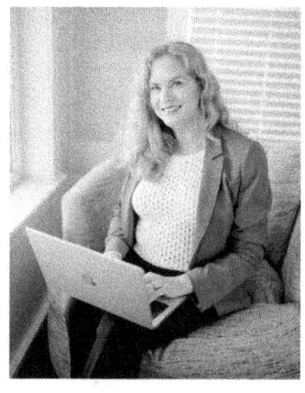

Before having both knees replaced and becoming "bionic," **Diana Braun** had a successful career in sales and marketing.

Diana took everything she learned about how to avoid, prepare for, and recover from knee replacement surgery and co-founded The Knee Zone with her husband, Dr. Sinha. She helps others by leading a free online education group, coaching, consulting, and speaking to groups around the country about knee replacement by leveraging her skills as a Certified High Performance Coach (CHPC).

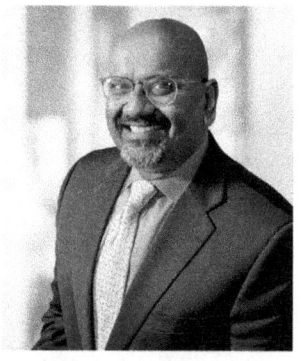

Raj Sinha, MD, PhD, is a board-certified orthopedic surgeon with more than 35 years of experience in Total Joint Replacement. He also has experience in academic medicine, private practice, surgeon education, hip and knee implant design, and clinical and basic science research.

Dr. Sinha enjoys exploring new solutions to age-old questions.

He cares for his patients like they are family. "The quality of care I want for my family and my mom and dad is exactly what I want to give to my patients every day," he says.

He tried retiring, but it didn't take—he missed helping patients too much. He's back in practice in Killeen, Texas.

Raj and Diana reside in Texas, where they golf and look after Karma, their entertaining dog. They enjoy building a community to help others learn about knee care.

MAY WE ASK A FAVOR?

If you enjoyed *Knee Replacements Secrets* and found it helpful, would you write an honest review and post it online?

It would mean the world to us!

Reviews are the best way to spread the word, reach more people, and help others avoid, plan for, or recover from knee replacement surgery.

Your Amazon, Goodreads, or social media recommendation could make a huge difference for someone who **knee'ds** this book.

Thank you!

HOW TO GET MORE HELP

Did *Knee Replacement Secrets* open your eyes to the options you "kneed'ed"?

As a bonus, schedule your free 15-minute private consultation with Diana.

You can ask her anything about her experience and learn more about working with **The Knee Zone** in a group or privately.

Simply scan the QR code below or visit:

TheKneeZone.com/consultation

www.ingramcontent.com/pod-product-compliance
Lightning Source LLC
Chambersburg PA
CBHW070621030426
42337CB00020B/3872